Secure accommodation in child care

Between hospital and prison or thereabouts?

Robert Harris and Noel Timms

ROUTLEDGE

London and New York

First published in 1993
by Routledge
11 New Fetter Lane, London EC4P 4EE

Simultaneously published in the USA and Canada
by Routledge
29 West 35th Street, New York, NY 10001

Typeset in 10/12 pt Times by LaserScript Limited, Mitcham, Surrey
Printed and bound in Great Britain by
Mackays of Chatham PLC, Chatham, Kent

British Library Cataloguing in Publication Data

A catalogue record for this book is available from the British Library.

Library of Congress Cataloging in Publication Data

Harris, Robert, 1947–
Secure accommodation in child care: 'between hospital and prison or thereabouts?'/Robert Harris and Noel Timms.
p. cm.
Includes bibliographical references and index.
1. Juvenile detention homes – Great Britain. 2. Social work with juvenile delinquents – Great Britain. I. Timms, Noel. II. Title.
HV9145.A5H367 1993
365′.42′0941 – dc20 92-38923
CIP

ISBN 0-415-06281-0
0-415-06282-9 (pbk)

Contents

Prologue vii
Acknowledgements xi

Part I Theoretical background: history, literature and social theory

1 Secure accommodation outlined 3

2 The state, the family and the child: a theoretical analysis 20

3 Young devils . . . or angels with dirty faces? 49

Part II Secure accommodation: some themes and issues from an empirical study

4 Talking to the experts 75

5 Secure children? 102

6 Insecure accommodations: the judicial hearings 138

7 What is to be done? 160

Appendix A: Child Care Act 1980, section 21A 173

Appendix B: Children Act 1989, section 25 175

Appendix C: Extract from the Criminal Justice Act 1991, section 60 177

Notes 179
Bibliography 183
Name index 191
Subject index 194

Prologue

> A man I knew from France . . . said to me once, rather happily: 'France, you know, is a bad bourgeois novel.' I could see how far he was right: the modes of dramatisation, of fictionalisation, which are active as social and cultural conventions, as ways not only of seeing but of organising reality, are as he said: a bourgeois novel . . . . 'Well yes', I said politely, 'England's a bad bourgeois novel too. And New York is a bad metropolitan novel. But there's one difficulty, at least I find it a difficulty. You can't send them back to the library. You're stuck with them. You have to read them over and over.' 'But critically,' he said, with an engaging alertness. 'Still reading them,' I said.
>
> (Williams 1975: 17–18)

This book grew out of a piece of research, but is not primarily a research report, seeking rather to use the subject of the research – secure accommodation in the child-care system – as a basis for a piece of social analysis, a case study in the relations of state, family (especially the deviant family) and child. It is a serious and sometimes complex book, but capable of being read at more than one level. Indeed it is integral to our purpose that this is so, for our audience will, we know, be diverse both professionally and academically. Our subject matter is difficult children, and how courts and professionals, in particular social workers, make decisions about them.

In order to make the book of value to professional readers, many of whom will be concerned with day-to-day issues surrounding the management of difficult children in difficult situations, we hope to paint a picture which both resonates with and clarifies their experiences, which articulates some of their dilemmas and helps them to work in a more reflective way. For policy makers, both at central and local government level, we hope to make some helpful suggestions. For social theorists, we hope to have broken new ground in our analysis of this particular corner of the relationship of state, family and child.

To address these various audiences competently requires the book to draw, at least in part, on the reformist tradition of policy and practice. It will become clear from our theoretical approach, however, that our habitation of this territory is somewhat equivocal. It is primarily (though by no means exclusively) to our more academically inclined readers that we address our equivocations, and for them that we identify the more theoretical meanings which emerge from the discourse within which this book is situated. For our enquiry will take us also into the more critical traditions of narrative, semiotics, postmodernism and post-structuralism, traditions which, though by no means new in themselves, are unusual accompaniments to a study of social policy and social work (though for examples of more tentative feints into some of these spheres, see Rojek *et al.* 1988, 1989).

To address multiple audiences is by no means necessarily to write a multiplicity of books, though like all but the most simple texts this one inhabits, as we all do, a world of paradox, ambiguity and contradiction. Certainly there are times when our theoretical analysis serves as an ironic gloss on our reformist aspirations, but at other times we hope that the imperative of relevance ensures that any Promethean tendencies remain incipient. Though complete integration of our perspectives is impossible, situating them in dialectical coexistence should be feasible; certainly the forms of knowledge we utilise are themselves interrelated. Since some parts of our analysis, including the 'accounts' of secure accommodation provided by professionals and children alike, are also intrinsically interesting and sometimes moving, we hope that this book, though sometimes complex, will be useful and stimulating for a wide range of readers.

The view which is occasionally expressed, at least in the field of social work (even on occasion by reviewers), that if a book cannot be understood easily by a busy (and by implication distracted) practitioner while eating a sandwich in the staff room it is probably not worth the effort, seems to us highly questionable. That complexity is sometimes manufactured by supposed experts, either for reasons of professional imperialism or, less insidiously and more simply, through linguistic infelicity, is beyond question; but to suggest that all complexity is of these kinds is philistine. The necessity or otherwise of our own more complex passages is, however, for readers, not authors, to determine.

Quantitatively, secure accommodation is but a small part of a large field. While up and down the country hundreds of thousands of children pass annually through the hands of social workers, only a few hundred find themselves, in the words of other researchers in this field, 'locked up' (Millham *et al.* 1978) in secure accommodation. As we wrestled with the ambiguities of secure accommodation, however, we came to appreciate that to study a small subject is not necessarily to be arcane or irrelevant. Just as, in the semiology which we shall encounter later, signifiers derive their meaning not from their intrinsic properties but from their relations to the sign system as a whole, so does secure accommodation derive meaning and logic from, and impart meaning and logic to, the whole complex relation of state, family and individual. If secure accommodation were not there, these relations would, in significant ways, be different.

This is both a general theoretical point and indicative of a particular trait of secure accommodation, something of the flavour of which is to be found in our sub-title (for the basis of which an anonymous professional respondent is to be thanked). Hospitals treat the sick, prisons hold the culpable; and secure accommodation, as we shall see, holds some youngsters said to be 'sick', some said to be 'wicked', some said to be both and some whom nobody seems to think are either but who do not quite fit in anywhere else.

The functions of secure accommodation, though legally ascribed, are analytically and professionally ambiguous, and much of what follows derives from this ambiguity. To 'lock up' children by means of an authorised strategy which embraces both 'sick' and 'wicked' is to suggest the existence of an interesting and less than obvious relation between meeting 'needs', furthering 'interests' and protecting 'rights', and to signal much about contemporary views on adolescent development, the nature of family and childhood, and juvenile crime.

There is also the intriguing ambiguity of the very concept 'secure'. Who (or what) are the subject and predicate of security? Is its purpose to provide an insecure youngster with psychological 'security', to provide the rest of us – adults and children alike – with 'security' from the youngster, or both? To some it is the former; to others of more cynical bent the latter, albeit sometimes disguised as the former, and with the secondary purpose of meeting the self-aggrandising demands of the child-care professionals as they engage in the endless pursuit of ever more children in need of their expertise and, in consequence, ever more resources.

We shall present a more complex picture. While not disagreeing with either of the most authoritative texts in our field (Millham *et al.* 1978; Cawson and Martell 1979) that subterfuge and aggrandisement exist (doubtless they flourish here as in all walks of life), we shall question whether these are sufficient conditions to explain both the usage and expansion of secure accommodation. We shall argue in the first three chapters that the dualistic mode of analysis – that secure accommodation is to be viewed *either* as benign and therapeutic *or* as cynical and covert oppression – is itself the product of a particular culture at a particular historical moment, and that to have a more rounded understanding of secure accommodation we must examine not only secure accommodation itself, not only child care, not only the relation between state and family, but also how all these together are understood in contemporary culture. It is not that the contemporary state cares for children *or* protects society; clearly it does both. The more interesting question is how the resulting practice of child care is understood and managed by the key actors in the drama. To understand that in turn, we must acknowledge and penetrate the official 'ideologies'[1] of childhood, family and state in order to discover how people make sense of their worlds. This, for reasons which will become clear, will take us into the world of literary and cultural theory, and in particular that of narrative.[2]

More questions follow. Supposing secure accommodation were abolished: what impact would this have on the rest of the child-care system? Would it contribute, as some reformers suggest, to a withdrawal of state control, or only to its displacement? The importance of questions such as these transcends the 'mere' issue of a disposal affecting a few hundred children a year, and it is matters of this kind which are addressed in this book. We begin by setting the scene in terms of history, law and social policy, providing the information necessary to make sense of what follows. In Chapter 2 we offer a brief revisionist history of the family, introducing a number of new concepts, including the key one of mythology.[3] Chapter 3, which draws the first, theoretical, part of the book to a close, develops a further theme – the use of forms of literary theory, notably narrative and drama – to help us further our enquiry.

The second part of the book then relates these theoretical ideas to the empirical study of secure accommodation. In Chapters 4 and 5 we report selected elements of our study of secure accommodation, focusing on the recorded transcripts of interviews about secure accommodation conducted with senior managers, professional workers and children. In Chapter 6 we report our observations of juvenile courts in action, determining whether or not local authorities shall be authorised to hold children in secure accommodation; and from this we distil a number of conclusions, some theoretical and some practical, which we present in Chapter 7. That we do not reproduce there all the twenty-six recommendations of our original research report is significant: time has moved on, some of our suggestions have come to pass, others have been overtaken by events. And, to reiterate our first sentence, this is not a research report, but a recasting into a new and we hope illuminating theoretical and conceptual framework of some of what we learned in the course of our work. Accordingly, for the most part Chapter 7 reflects what we report here, not the totality of the research; but we believe it to be significant none the less, and hope it is interesting.

Acknowledgements

Many friends and colleagues, none of whom bears responsibility for this book's final form, have helped and advised us in its preparation. Particular thanks are due to Ms Mary Henkel of the Department of Government, Brunel University; Mrs Rita Timms, formerly of the Values Centre, University of Leicester; Ms Kathy Laster of the Department of Criminology, University of Melbourne; Mrs Linda Burnham, Guardian *ad litem*, Hull; and, by no means least, to the first author's colleagues at the University of Hull: Dr Subrata Mitra of the Department of Politics, Mr Martin Parry of the Law School, and Dr Marion Shaw of the Department of English.

Thanks are also due to the Department of Health and Social Security (as it then was) for funding the empirical research on which the book is based, and, within the Department, to a number of officials, in particular Dr Carolyn Davies and Mr Bryan Hopper, for their advice throughout. Our gratitude to the children and professionals we interviewed is none the less genuine for being necessarily non-specific; and the study could not have been completed without the efforts of our research officer Ms Siân Parry, and the sessional researchers hired to observe the juvenile court hearings.

Part I

Theoretical background

History, literature and social theory

1 Secure accommodation outlined

> In the war waged by the State against irregular families . . . the child is no more than a pretext and a hostage. Parental authority is an instrument distributed by the State, which the State consequently has the power to retract. The absolute weapon of those who inspect how families run their lives is to take away, or threaten to take away, the children. All children who are 'guilty' or 'unhappy' or 'irregular' or 'neglected', to use the expressions most current in the mouths of philanthropists, come from a poorly kept family.
>
> (Meyer 1983: 11–12)

> What we've never done is give the opportunity for children to stay in secure accommodation without a secure order, which is an interesting way to use it.
>
> (Interviewee)

SECURE ACCOMMODATION: AMBIGUITY IN ACTION

Secure accommodation is available to, and normally provided by, local authorities for use in respect of three main categories of youngster: children[1] committed to care,[2] those remanded awaiting trial or sentence[3] and those serving sentences of detention under the Children and Young Persons Act 1933 (section 53). We shall have more to say about these youngsters later.

Since 1983, in order to hold a youngster in secure accommodation for more than 72 hours in any 28-day period a local authority has had to obtain an authorisation from a juvenile court (see Appendix A). Prior to this there existed few restrictions on local authorities' use of such accommodation, and our research was commissioned to study the impact of the new legislation on the practices of local authorities. At the time of the study an authorisation could be granted on one of two main grounds: briefly, that the child, having a history of absconding, was likely to abscond again and, if he did so, was likely to put his physical, mental or moral welfare at risk;[4] or that the child, if not kept in secure accommodation, was likely to harm himself or others. The length of time a child may be held in secure accommodation is specified by regulation; then as now it was 3 months at a first hearing and 6 months on renewal.

In spite of occasional appearances to the contrary, an authorisation is not a sentence; indeed the local authority is not empowered to hold a youngster in secure accommodation once the circumstances which led to the making of the authorisation have ceased to exist: the 3- and 6-month periods are maxima, and early release is formally encouraged. As we shall see later, however, things are not so simple in practice.

Secure accommodation is a fundamentally ambiguous facility, and to view it in isolation from the much larger child-care and delinquency systems of which it is a part is to miss both the nature and significance of this ambiguity. Secure accommodation is both incarceration and an alternative to incarceration, a form of control imposed in order that care can be provided. This has certain ramifications, all of which suggest the likelihood of continuing pressure to expand the system. Politically, as a humane form of custody with therapeutic aspirations it has an attractiveness to both the liberal rehabilitative and the conservative law and order lobbies; professionally, by embracing both youngsters who would otherwise be in less pleasant institutions and those who would otherwise be in open conditions it has created pressure for more 'experts', better trained and with enhanced influence and status. In secure accommodation the penal and the therapeutic, the controlling and the caring converge, and the resulting ambiguity is central to the system's logic. Secure accommodation is the point at which the protection of children and the protection of others against those same children merge into a single carceral disposal.[5]

Ambiguity presents problems and opportunities for both policy makers and front-line professional workers, and the rules of engagement derive ultimately from the fact that secure accommodation seeks to address three contested issues, all of them intrinsically complex as well as controversial – those of needs, rights and interests. The necessity of maintaining an equilibrium among these concepts, affording sovereignty to none, means that the conventional attempt to eliminate ambiguity by rule making can only take us so far. For not only are rules regularly ignored or manipulated by those subject to them, but they are by nature general, while each 'case' is unique, with its own combination of characteristics seldom amenable to simple or routine interventions: applying general rules to specific cases necessitates discretion, for there is seldom only one possible answer. This point is accentuated when a single disposition is required, as this one is, to engage with concepts which, if unyoked from each other, would take us in quite different directions. Accordingly as we progress we shall see that attempts to use secure accommodation solely within a framework of rights *or* needs *or* interests is by no means to simplify but to be simplistic.

Obviously ambiguity is by no means unique to secure accommodation. Because it facilitates strategic and flexible policy implementation it is indispensable to many penal disposals (Harris and Webb 1987: 163), other social policies (Harris 1990) and indeed the interpretation of statute generally (Zander 1980: ch. 2). In criminal justice it reflects the belief that there is seldom a 'right' sentence in a given case, and allows for changes in circumstance during the course of the disposal. Both community service orders and the range of prisons, from 'open'[6] establishments on the South coast to dungeon-like institutions in remote corners of northern England, provide just this form of manoeuvrability: the finer a system's calibrations the greater its utility (Cohen 1985; Harris and Webb 1987).[7] The calibrations both build in a legitimate and necessary role for experts (who inevitably determine these fraught allocations) and create a logical system of rewards and punishments as individuals are, on the basis of their conduct and response to treatment, moved along the continuum of harshness and care. This in turn transforms the sentence from an event into a process, a site for a succession of determinations influenced less by the original crime than by the subsequent behaviour of the criminal.

Secure accommodation, in embracing not only different categories of offender but also non-offenders, seeks simultaneously to meet the needs of disturbed or unfortunate youngsters and to inject discipline and structure into the lives of the deviant young. For secure accommodation is precisely the locus in which the question of whether a child has committed an offence or is in some other way problematic ceases to matter. And the decisiveness of this expression of the state's interest in the realm of family and childhood deviance teaches us much both about the state and about its management of families and children. This is why, if we are to understand secure accommodation, we cannot examine secure accommodation alone. This first chapter, therefore, provides both basic information about the system and some of the analytic equipment necessary to enable us to complete our journey in reasonable shape.

At the most abstract level, extracted from their historical, social, political, administrative and cultural contexts, the words 'secure' and 'accommodation' are of course meaningless. Even if we concede a general area of shared understanding – that 'secure accommodation' is an amalgam of the name given to certain categories of buildings of containment and the laws which permit that containment – the 'meaning' of such buildings and such laws derives both from the social purpose of holding children in this way and from the manner in which the holding relates to other options available.

The taken-for-granted assumption that there must *be* secure accommodation arises from certain historical trends in child-care policy. In a long historical perspective these have involved the gradual *distancing* of provisions for juvenile offenders and adult criminals, and the complementary *merging* of facilities for delinquents and needy children (Heywood 1978; Packman 1981; Harris and Webb 1987). These shifts have not always been smooth; they too have about them an ambiguity acknowledging the awkward coexistence of deprivation and malevolence, for the misbehaviour of the young is conventionally regarded as a blend of personal or social misery and deliberate crime, and the social response to delinquency must accordingly involve the coexistence of the notions that crime is the product of external social forces and that it is deliberately chosen. The fates may not have dealt a good hand to many of the children who concern us in this book, but in contemporary political discourse the children are none the less blameworthy for succumbing to temptation.

JUVENILE DELINQUENCY: THEMES AND ISSUES

Until the early nineteenth century there was no readily available concept of juvenile delinquency. This is not to deny that youngsters committed crimes, that the period we would now term 'adolescence' was perceived to be 'difficult', that there existed humane judges, or that day-to-day accommodations were made to what was, then as now, perceived as the immaturity of youth. It is rather to argue that since 'juvenile delinquency' was not of a distinctive form no specific strategies had been created to deal with it.

Such strategies began in mid-century, stemming, depending on our approach to history, from the efforts of individual 'great men (or in this case women) of history' who by passion, commitment and eloquence swayed nations to their point of view; from a collective humane concern about the social costs of industrialisation; or from the class interests of the mercantile bourgeoisie in stemming the threat of revolution which had materialised in many countries in continental Europe between 1789 and 1848, and in creating a compliant labour force for the mills and factories. As our own story unfolds, however, it will become apparent that to us none of these encapsulated ideas adequately embraces the inchoate nature of the social understanding of, and response to, the amalgam of youthful experience and behaviour which we term 'delinquency'. For this book does not posit policy development as linear and progressive, with the state moving inexorably towards greater rationality, efficiency or humanity. Our image, on the contrary, is of the various arms of an anything but monolithic state grappling as best they can, first with the often unanswerable problems posed by deviant and distressed children and secondly with the unintended consequences of their own earlier and unsuccessful endeavours.

Before the 'creation' of juvenile delinquency there existed conceptually distinct categories of childhood need and adult crime. The crucial contribution of the concept juvenile delinquency to understanding each was that it bridged the two. Juvenile delinquency, though in contemporary discourse it is used synonymously with 'juvenile crime', refers, literally, to 'neglect of duty', and involves simultaneously addressing on the one hand immaturity and deprivation, and on the other criminality, all of these being inextricably intertwined in the small person of the child. And it is essential to understand that the carceral structures created as a response to juvenile delinquency are not mere responses to it but central aspects of the social construction of the concept itself (Foucault 1977). To have been a 'provie [approved school] boy' or a 'Borstal boy' is to carry a signification not only of the institution in which one happens to have been contained but of one's own characteristics, experiences and conduct. Hence:

> The delinquent is not the author of a criminal act pure and simple, rather the delinquent is a life, a collection of biographical details and psychological characteristics. The delinquent is also 'an object' in a field of knowledge, a field patrolled by experts – jurists, but also psychologists, social workers, in short a whole series of professional biographers, whose task has been to change the reference point of criminality from the act to the life.
>
> (Boyne 1990: 116)

This intertwining has complicated the notions of both childhood and crime (see, for example, Bailey 1987), creating policy problems to which secure accommodation constitutes one attempted solution. So our image of 'childhood' carries traces of self-seeking voluntarism *and* helplessness or immaturity; the child cries out both to be socialised *and* to be loved. And though lower-class children in particular may experience disadvantage and pain they have opportunities too, which they must be encouraged to grasp. It is in part in furtherance of this that the state's functions turn both on meeting needs and interests and on protecting rights. When, however, the helping hand of the benign state is spurned and the crimes continue, persuasion and control become necessary. While this does not make the benignity of the state a fraud, it endows it with a certain conditionality, rendering it, perhaps, a clause in an individually renegotiated social contract: the state gives more to the child, but in return expects more back.

The child delinquent, therefore, is to be punished yet helped, and in varying proportions depending on the nature of the 'case' as determined by law and professional opinion. Nor, however, can the family which, both responsible and not responsible, culpable and not culpable, plays a complex role, be left outside of this process: while it is over the child that the court stands in judgment, the judgment is of a particular and qualified kind which by no means excludes the possibility of advising or rebuking the parents. While allowances are made because, had the child had better parents he or she would not be in trouble, the existence of bad parents is of itself insufficient justification for delinquency. How else, therefore, is the state to respond but by an amalgam of care and control directed not solely at the child but at the family too? However complex in practice sustaining such a duality may be, analytically it is difficult to see how else to proceed.

These seemingly contradictory responses to the delinquent child have different historical traces. We are carriers of successive 'dominant' views of history, cumulatively not substitutively, and these views coalesce to 'create' today's images of childhood. These images are not simple, and we must avoid the trap of believing that we have an agreed 'image of childhood' which guides our actions and beliefs. First, except in the case of very young children we seldom regard the child as qualitatively different from the adult; secondly, we do not regard children of all ages as homogeneous in the way that we may conceive, say, of a 'responsible' adult; thirdly, we cannot decide how to determine whether and to what extent children can exercise the responsibilities and discharge the obligations of citizenship (Harris, J. 1982); and fourthly, we tend to regard 'childhood' as a voyage, a form of progress towards the threshold of maturity. Hence it is 'obvious' that the 15-year-old should be more mature than the 10-year-old in a way that it is not 'obvious' that a 35-year-old should be more mature than a 30-year-old. The mutability of childhood, which contrasts so strikingly with the relative stasis of adulthood (at least until the onset of old age), offers a bewildering and contradictory array of images on which to draw in a particular 'case'. So complex is this activity indeed that it can only be undertaken by experts, whose selection and application of explanatory theories are prerequisites for authoritative judgements (Harris and Webb 1987: ch. 2).

This is, of course, very much a twentieth-century perspective from which to view the nineteenth century's nascent attempts to create structures to address this phenomenon of delinquency. In spite of piecemeal attempts to distinguish the treatment of young from that of adult offenders in the early years of the last century (Harris and Webb 1987: 10–11), it was reformatory and industrial schools, instituted in the 1850s, which were the most significant developments, signifying as they did the more systematic segregation of young and adult offenders. Reformatory schools, for Mary Carpenter's designated 'dangerous classes', received legislative sanction in the Youthful Offenders Act 1854, quickly becoming the standard disposal for a second offence (though always following a period of hard labour, in order both that punishment was inflicted and that the child arrived suitably chastened). Industrial schools were initially for those 'at risk' non-offenders designated the 'perishing classes' (Carpenter 1851; see also Manton 1976).

We see in this realignment of adult criminals, juvenile criminals and needy children only an interim stage in the reconceptualisation of delinquency which has since occurred. The creation of reforming institutions for youthful offenders and, separately from that, of corrective institutions for the wayward pre-delinquent constitutes an acknowledgement of the 'separateness' of adult and young offenders but not yet of the relative interchangeability of the dangerous and perishing classes. The inadequacies of this division, however, quickly became manifest. The perishing classes contained many vagrants, a group which, because they would not stay 'placed', had traditionally worried the ruling classes. One contemporary account noted that two-thirds of London criminals had 'migratory habits' (Day 1858: 76; see also Tobias 1972: ch. 5; and Priestley 1985: 57), and the removal of street children who seemed at once miserable and threatening was attractive both to the self-interested bourgeoisie and to the reforming conscience. The Industrial Schools Act was passed in 1857 and steadily extended, notably in 1866 and 1908, by which time was permitted the commitment of children aged 7 to 14 who were vagrant, begging, destitute because their parents were serving penal servitude, under the care of a drunken or criminal guardian, frequenting the company of reputed thieves or prostitutes or residing in premises used for prostitution.

Though provisions of this kind were not new, and it may indeed be that the idea of industrial schools is 'as old as the poor law' (Rose 1967: 4), the second half of the nineteenth century, in which industrial schools were holding some 15,000 children at any one time, remains the apotheosis of the attempt at the institutional socialisation of the young. A trade-off began to occur between unpleasantness and length of sentence, and so great was political confidence in the reformatory school system that by the end of the century even the short periods of pre-reformatory hard labour were abolished (Reformatory Schools Amendment Act 1899). All sentences of imprisonment on children were abolished by the Children Act 1908.

Both kinds of school were involved, with largely interchangeable children, in the enterprise of training them for the factory or domestic labour for which they were normally destined. Both operated, more through administrative convenience than theoretical purism, regimes based on uniformity; both emphasised the merits of absolute conformity; both were strongly driven by the imperative of religious instruction; both, ironically given Mary Carpenter's loathing of the Parkhurst experiment, resembled nothing so much as the prison – as though there were no other model on which their operations could be based. Both reformatory and industrial schools sought to resocialise the deviant or potentially deviant young by long-term correctional placement, and the sanction given the schools signified the state's determination to intervene actively in the lives of children not only as they would in those of adults – as a response to crime – but in a manner which reflected the particular economic and social 'value' of childhood.

Hence the introduction of reformatory and industrial schools signified a rupture of the assumption that juvenile crime was simply a modified form of adult crime, though there was as yet little conception of an alternative framework by means of which to comprehend 'delinquency'. No formalised discipline of psychology yet existed to explain the existence of this new and ambiguous form of deviance, and the notion of 'difference' could therefore be couched only in that sphere of theologically driven humanitarianism which existed, in a pre-Freudian era, in the space later to be occupied by the analytic, developmental, cognitive, moral, social and behavioural psychologies. The more significant shifts occurred, therefore, with the new political and economic value which, from the final years of the nineteenth century, came to be attached to childhood. This was reflected penologically in the move away from theories of uniformity towards individualisation (Gladstone Report 1895) and continued in the child welfare legislation of the Asquith administration (1906–14) with its introduction of the School Medical Service, school meals, health visitors, probation, Borstal training, juvenile courts and the prohibition of cigarette sales to, and the imprisonment of, children.

Significantly, it was this era too when a new ambiguity again became manifest. The simple distinction between dangerous and perishing classes had proved unsustainable by the end of the century, and industrial schools legislation began increasingly to include younger thieves in these schools, partly to prevent *them* from being contaminated by the more sophisticated of the reformatory schoolchildren and partly for administrative convenience (Rose 1967). More significant still was an official report of 1896 which, in arguing that there was no significant difference in the regimes of, or in the children held in, the two kinds of school (*Report of the Departmental Committee on Reformatory and Industrial Schools* 1896), initiated a process culminating in the merging of the schools themselves in the Children and Young Persons Act 1933.

This process was hastened further by the decline in the usage of these facilities following the introduction of compulsory education, the expansion of the Probation Service and increasing objections by penal reformers such as the Howard Association (Bochel 1976: 15) and influential magistrates (Clarke Hall 1926: 142) to over-dependence on institutions. Some courts, to government consternation, had taken to using reformatory and industrial schools interchangeably with the conditions of residence which could be attached to probation orders, and the ensuing reductions in the usage of the schools, combined with official acceptance that probation supervision was suitable for non-delinquent as well as delinquent children (Departmental Committee Report 1927), meant that the continuation of a dual system was neither defensible nor practicable.

Home Office Approved Schools, for offenders and non-offenders alike, came into being following the implementation of the Children and Young Persons Act 1933. This Act, the first to lay upon the courts the obligation to 'have regard for the welfare of the child or young person' (section 44), reduced the maximum period of commitment from five years to three, but extended the range of youngsters liable to commitment both in age and problem category (Harris and Webb 1987: 16). Cases where the 'welfare of the child' would best be met by the institution were now eligible for Approved Schools as were children categorised as 'beyond control', a clause subjected to contemporary criticism for supposedly relieving neglectful parents of responsibility for their family (Page 1936: 192–3).

The Act blurred the boundaries of need and punishment in child care. Its emphasis on 'welfare', however, inevitably led to the containment of many needy non-delinquents (particularly girls) in facilities also used for offenders; and its inclusion of 'beyond control' children signified a shift in state involvement in child care from the relatively marginal to the central. The legislation made the effective control of the children a new condition to be met by families if they were to be permitted to keep them at home. Every step the state takes to concern itself with the upbringing of the child is an intimation of its willingness to exercise control of a kind the families themselves have been unable or unwilling to demonstrate. When the state ceases to turn a blind eye to misery, deviance or self-harm, increasingly decisive forms of control become necessary to deal with problems which have defeated the best efforts of others.

The detailed changes in juvenile justice of the 1960s leading to the Children and Young Persons Act 1969 have been fully described elsewhere (Harris, R. 1982; Harris and Webb 1987: 22–31) and are not recapitulated here. For our present theme three points suffice. First, the 1969 Act created an administrative structure which unified provisions for young offenders with those for needy children in the belief that to do so would lead to a liberalisation of the social response to the former. This administrative unification, however, seriously under-estimated the political and cultural significance of the single obvious difference between offenders and non-offenders – that the one group was being dealt with for a crime while the other was not; and it was in particular not accompanied by any conceptual, theoretical or moral structure signifying that criminality was 'externally' caused. The procedures, therefore, provoked widespread criticism, and were subverted by the most significant actors in the drama, magistrates, police and justices' clerks.

Secondly, partly in consequence of this subversion, a large increase in institutional sentencing occurred, sometimes on interchangeable therapeutic and punitive grounds; and thirdly, the 'blurring of the boundaries' led not only to the destigmatisation of offenders but to the simultaneous and consequential stigmatisation of those needy children now correctly perceived as largely interchangeable with them. These factors in turn created political pressure from both liberals and conservatives (though for different reasons), to reduce institutional sentencing, an objective which became a major feature of the penal policy of the 1980s (Harris 1991).

SECURE ACCOMMODATION: THE HISTORICAL BACKGROUND

Approved Schools were 'open' facilities introduced when the crime rate was relatively low and most serious young offenders committed to Borstal. With the main exception of absconding (Franklin Report 1951; Clarke and Martin 1971), the system operated fairly smoothly until well into the post-war period. The Curtis Report, for example, while deploring the tendency to regimentation and lack of feminine influence in some of the boys' schools, pronounced them generally 'well conducted in a humane and experimental spirit' (*Report of the Care of Children Committee* 1946: para. 499). By the early 1960s, however, this tranquillity was being disturbed both by an increasing crime rate and by a new politicality attaching to juvenile crime. The 'open' structures were increasingly defied by trainees, and by the mid-1960s a policy problem had emerged to which there existed as yet no solution:

> a number of these boys ought to be kept for a time at least in closed conditions – anathema to most approved school staff – and it is only recently that closed blocks have been attached to the classifying schools. In other systems, such as borstal, where the security risk is an integral element of allocation and of the training system, a closed block for 'cooling off' and re-allocation is provided for boys removed from their institutions.
>
> (Rose 1967: 52)

The post-war era saw a significant shift in the usage of closed institutions which were now only partially concerned with the punishment or training of the serious criminal, increasingly becoming the 'hard end' of an integrated system embracing juvenile justice *and* child care, with the task of holding youngsters who had proved too difficult for open establishments (Cawson and Martell 1979: 4). Community homes were variegated, enabling transfers to take place between facilities primarily for the distressed and those primarily for the criminal, and for all the liberal rhetoric the administration of justice and child-care facilities was concerned less with ontological questions of human behaviour than with effective management. To introduce an administrative approach which blurs the boundaries between social need and crime is not to attribute aetiological significance to either but to create a framework into which both the 'needy' and the 'delinquent' can be inserted and manipulated by executive adjudication. To blur boundaries no more 'abolishes' juvenile delinquency than it 'abolishes' need, a point not lost on a magistrate referred to by one of our interviewees:

> The Chairperson of the Bench wrote to express concern. There was one child admitted here that she felt was wrongly admitted – not to secure (though he ended up there actually) he was admitted to this building and she wrote asking why and expressing concern that a care kid had been put in with all the criminals and we'd turn him into a criminal.

The motif is not the encapsulation of one by the other but the generation of a new, synthetic, concept, bounded neither by 'need' nor 'criminality' but, because it embraces both, paradoxically different from either. We do not have a word for this concept other than 'delinquency', and this, in spite of its etymology, is too often used synonymously with 'youthful criminality' to embrace our meaning.

As the Approved School system in the 1950s changed its clientele and hence its image, absconding became a more serious problem (see, for example, Maxwell 1956; Slater 1967). This led to a recommendation by the Children's Department Inspectorate that 'closed blocks' should be attached to specified Approved Schools and decisions for transfer made, as ever, on the basis of different considerations:

> the needs of the boy, of the outside community, and of the open school were to be examined, but there was no discussion of the possibility that these might on occasion be in conflict, or decision on which should have priority.
>
> (Cawson and Martell 1979: 6)

The consideration being given to closed blocks received a new impetus from serious disturbances in 1959 at Carlton Approved School, the report of an enquiry into which (*Report of the Enquiry into the Disturbances at*

Carlton School in August 1959) attributed responsibility to a combination of poor staff–boy relations and to the fact that the calibre of boys being admitted was deteriorating. This report recommended the adoption of secure units in some schools on a regional basis, detention rooms in all schools and the transfer to Borstal of disruptive elements. A Home Office Report which appeared shortly afterwards (*Report of the Home Office Working Party on Closed and Other Special Facilities in Approved Schools* 1960) recommended attaching closed blocks to classifying schools, as did a third report, this time organised by the Approved Schools Central Advisory Committee Working Party but chaired by a Home Office representative. To the sceptics, ever in search of classificatory precision,

> the units were to be a rag-bag of those boys who were disrupting the system, a function that was to be extended as new categories of threatening adolescents were created. For example, children who committed very serious crimes (Section 53 of the Children and Young Persons Act 1933) were added in 1968 and boys with threatening homosexual behaviour in 1969. Treatment, even if known, could hardly be applied to such a varied group of children.
>
> (Millham *et al.* 1978: 25)

The first of the regional special units recommended by the Carlton enquiry report opened at Kingswood Classifying School, Bristol, in 1964, followed by Redhill in 1965 and Redbank in 1966. Increasingly, however, monitoring of the system began to identify a gap between rehabilitative rhetoric and therapeutic practice as professional power and interests moved inexorably to fill that vacuum which exists in any administrative corollary of an ambiguous or intractable problem: 'Instead of admitting boys for a short period of six months, and then returning them to open schools, the units were developing complete treatment programmes of their own, keeping boys until the time of their discharge' (Cawson and Martell 1979: 17). Staff defended this practice by 'stating the advantages of continuity of care and relationships with staff, for boys who had such interrupted histories and problematic family relationships' (1979: 18), beginning to identify the units as proper sites for the therapy of youngsters who would otherwise 'run away', not only literally but psychologically, from themselves and their problems (Millham *et al.* 1978: 27). In the words of one of our own respondents, speaking of his own secure unit:

> There is also a basic philosophy that children who have been absconding have been using absconding as a means of avoiding looking at what has been going on. In secure we take away from them that option and they are then confronted with the problems and they haven't got the option of

> running away from them. They then have to develop another strategy of coping with them.

Heads of homes were empowered to regulate intakes by accepting or rejecting referrals, and because in consequence the more therapeutically attractive youngsters were more likely to be accepted than extraverted, intermittently violent ones, the system's logic was expansionist. The heads' rejection of the residual function of holding a small number of extremely difficult children meant that these youngsters would have to be contained elsewhere while the units busied themselves with their new target group of youngsters. These were youngsters who, for psychological reasons and against their own interests, would flee help when it was offered, youngsters for whom a humane and therapeutically inspired closed institution seemed tailor-made. The need was for both physical and psychological security, but so immense was the psychic damage done to these children that the task was likely to prove neither simple nor speedy.

This rejection of the most disruptive youngsters created pressure for super-secure units to deal with those additionally disturbed youngsters for whom the original units were devised, but whose problems were now deemed to require more specialist expertise. The idea emerged, encouraged in particular by the highly publicised case of a girl murderess for whom no suitable facility was available, of Regional Youth Treatment Centres, funded by central government but with charges levied on local authorities according to usage. As planning proceeded, however, the history of the special units began to repeat itself:

> while the Home Office Children's Department were concerned that there should be a unit available in which children could, if necessary, be detained in conditions of maximum security, the Working Party with its heavy balance of personnel from medical and child care professions, were planning to provide long term treatment, which would, however, involve only short term physical security in closed conditions.
>
> (Cawson and Martell 1979: 33–4)

The St Charles Youth Treatment Centre, with its psychoanalytically derived therapeutic regime, opened in Brentwood, Essex, in 1971; its behavioural counterpart, Glenthorne, followed in Erdington, Birmingham, in 1978. Plans for a third centre were not pursued.

Alongside the development of the YTCs was an exponential increase in local authority secure units in the 1970s, a move funded by capital grants from central government with almost unanimous support from the professionals concerned. This expansion was part of a more general trend of high institutional usage in a decade which saw a 500 per cent increase in the use of penal institutions (Department of Health and Social Security 1981b), and the regional planning of secure provision proceeded with little professional *Angst*. For example, with the sole exception of the pressure group Radical Alternatives to Prison, witnesses to the House of Commons Expenditure Committee in 1975 argued the inadequacy of the 200 secure places then available. Even the Howard League for Penal Reform (though characteristically also calling for more research) did not dissent from this expansionism, thereby finding itself, doubtless to its collective bewilderment, on the same side of the fence as the Police Federation and the Magistrates' Association: 'Most witnesses argued very strongly that more secure accommodation was needed . . . estimates of the total number of places needed varied from 600 suggested by the Regional Planning Committees to 2,500 recommended by the Residential Care Association' (House of Commons 1975: para. 72). The DHSS had, throughout most of the decade, provided the grants for which it was pressed, in spite of having no clear guidelines for considering applications. Though security was to be used only *in extremis* for the 'persistent absconder' and the 'intractable and anti-social' (Home Office 1960) these terms remained undefined, and a subsequent Circular, *Secure Accommodation in Community Homes* (Department of Health and Social Security 1975), equally lacked operational clarity. The policy emphasis at this time was neither on enhancing children's rights nor on decarceration (both to be major themes of the 1980s) but on mustering a case for increased public expenditure on ever more units and facilities, and on the increased training of ever more expert staff.

SECURE ACCOMMODATION: TOWARDS LEGISLATIVE CHANGE

By the middle of the 1970s a number of objections, to become increasingly audible by the end of the decade, were being expressed. First, there was questioning of the appropriateness of secure accommodation in dealing with absconding. The Expenditure Committee, in a paragraph not translated into a recommendation, had itself alluded approvingly to countries which

> take a more relaxed view of the problem of absconding than appears to be customary in England and Wales. Provided that a child shows some signs of improvement in other ways it is simply located and brought back if it runs away; in Sweden a case was quoted to us of a girl who had run away sixteen times and was still living in the establishment concerned. We do not consider that absconding in itself should result in a child being locked up.
>
> (House of Commons 1975: para. 78)

Secondly, concern was being expressed that less problematic youngsters were being held in security: that empty places were attracting users rather than being a response to shortages. We shall encounter this argument again later:

> the boys in the units at present are less problematic than they have ever been. . . a stay in certain community homes guarantees that disruptive conduct will lead to a recommendation for security and it is just as clear that similar conduct elsewhere will not.
>
> (Millham *et al.* 1978: 46–7)

Thirdly, the concept of children's 'rights', though theoretically and conceptually inchoate (for a flavour of which inchoation see, for example, Holt 1975), had begun to assume political and professional significance by about 1978. This had been fostered by the United Nations Year of the Child, as part of which was founded the Children's Legal Centre (Children's Legal Centre 1982, 1983; Harris 1991), and fanned by the appearance of *Who Cares?* (Page and Clark 1977), a booklet which contributed to the formation of the rights-based group the National Association of Young People in Care (see Franklin 1986).

The fourth emergent concern was with the importance of defining clear guidelines for the use of secure accommodation, the absence of which was assumed to have contributed to the variant uses of secure accommodation by local authorities. The two existing circulars (DHSS 1972, 1975) required updating, and a working group chaired by Barbara Kahan was convened to provide guidelines for the inspection of secure units (DHSS 1979). It noted how broad the criteria for admission to security had become: 'any child in care of any age or either sex may be admitted to secure accommodation if this is considered to be in his own interest or for the protection of other persons' (DHSS 1979: para. 8.4). By this time, fuelled by the dawning awareness that a major departure in child-care policy had emerged virtually unplanned, unmonitored and unevaluated, secure accommodation had become a significant issue in the internal politics of the DHSS. The economic crisis of the late 1970s brought home to all the spending departments the cost to the Exchequer of their policies, and the continued expansion of institutional care at the rate of the 1970s would have been impossible. A developing political attack on professional autonomy combined with a new stress on legalism paved the way for credence to be given to a legal lobby of 'rights' lawyers, and these processes augmented the pressure from some of the Department's own senior staff to restrain the discretionary powers of the child-care professionals.

Accordingly, in addition to the Kahan Report and the Department's own highly critical research (Cawson and Martell 1979), a third study was begun. A departmental working group chaired by Norman Tutt, whose members had access to both the Cawson and Martell and the Dartington studies, was enjoined to recommend how the use made of secure accommodation by local authorities should be structured (DHSS 1981a). Significantly, the working group recommended that in future a child should enter secure accommodation only by the *legal route* of a court authorisation, and no longer on executive discretion. Tutt argued that to incarcerate people without a court hearing was contrary to 'natural justice' and, more tangibly, in breach of Article 5.4 of the European Convention on Human Rights:

> Everyone who is deprived of his liberty on arrest or detention shall be entitled to take proceedings by which the lawfulness of his detention shall be decided speedily by a court and his release ordered if the detention is not lawful.

The Convention was topical at the time, since a case awaiting adjudication by the European Court, *X* v. *The United Kingdom*, turned on the legality of the executive detention of mental patients. Once this case had been resolved in favour of the complainant (in November 1981), the analogy with child care was such that the conclusion that existing arrangements for secure accommodation in the child-care system were contrary to European law became inescapable.

Though an adverse determination in the European Court of Justice seldom precipitates a speedy change in national law, the judgment signalled that secure accommodation had become what an informant closely involved in the debates of the time described to us as a 'winnable issue'. Key civil servants, the newly formed Children's Legal Centre, the Parliamentary All-Party Penal Affairs Committee and the National Association for the Care and Resettlement of Offenders (whose senior officer Paul Cavadino was secretary to the Penal Affairs Committee) began to mount a concerted political campaign which, had it been resisted, had the potential to create political embarrassment: a government which was reflecting critically on whether the continued existence of statutory social work itself was necessary would have found itself having to defend the principle that social workers should determine a question of children's liberty.

When the legislative change came it came quickly, with a rushed amendment to section 25 of the Criminal Justice Bill 1982 (and a further amendment, to correct a drafting error, to the Health and Social Services and Social Security Adjudications Bill 1983) by means of which a new section, 21A, was inserted into the Child Care Act 1980 (see Appendix A). The original amendment came into force in May 1983, and the revision in January 1984. The legislation was repealed in 1991 and replaced by the provisions of the Children Act 1989, section 25 (see Appendix B). We return to these detailed matters in Chapter 4.

CONCLUSION

Historically, secure accommodation has been an attempt to solve simultaneously both the problems created by deviant children who have resisted all gentler forms of persuasion and those of the needy and desperate child whose response to kindness is to run away. The security provided is psychological as well as physical, the help individualised, the care and concern of the staff doubtless genuine.

Secure accommodation, while not removing the problem of the difficult youngster, attempts to contain it. The persistently ambiguous characteristics of secure accommodation suggest that we are not in the simple domain of solving problems and maintaining solutions. Secure accommodation is a response to the insoluble, a space at which to take pause. If we do not wish to be neglectful of the needy child we take over some of the functions of parenting from the parents themselves; yet if we support the unsuccessful or recalcitrant families with help and resources we reward the very families which break the rules; but if we do not do so the children suffer. And in taking on these responsibilities to allow the children to whom that responsibility extends to run wild against our instructions is as clear a definition of bad parenting as we can conceive; yet if we prevent them from running by containing them compulsorily, how do we distinguish our proper social concern, both for them and for those others they may harm, from imprisonment?

This is a flavour of the dilemmas, paradoxes and contradictions with which a consideration of secure accommodation confronts us, and which help explain why our journey will be circuitous, why to understand secure accommodation alone is to understand little or nothing of why it exists, why it is so fraught and poignant an intervention.

2 The state, the family and the child

A theoretical analysis

> As a child he had heard vaguely about the notorious Yorkshire schools, and in particular he remembered the story of a 'suppurated abscess that some boy had come home with in consequence of his Yorkshire guide, philosopher and friend' – in other words, the schoolmaster – ' . . . having ripped it open with an inky pen-knife'. He remained 'curious' about these schools, which were in many instances nothing but convenient dustbins for unwanted children, bastards or orphans; the advertisements for them often included the chilling words, 'No Vacations', which meant that the children were retained there indefinitely.
>
> (Peter Ackroyd 1990: 249–50)

> Flaubert was a giant; they all said so. He towered over everybody like a strapping Gallic chieftain. And yet he was only six feet tall. . . the world shrinks just a little with that knowledge. The giants were not so tall (were the dwarfs therefore shorter too?). The fat men: were they less fat because they were smaller, and so you needed less stomach to appear fat; or were they more fat, because they developed the same stomachs, but had even less frame to support them? How can we know such trivial, crucial details? We can study files for decades, but every so often we are tempted to throw up our hands and declare that history is merely another literary genre: the past is autobiographical fiction pretending to be a parliamentary report.
>
> (Julian Barnes 1984: 90)

The interdependence of secure accommodation with all aspects of public child care has both spatial and temporal dimensions. Spatially it is variably used by different courts, agencies and regimes, all of which are in consequence actively defining and redefining the nature both of the primary deviance and of secure accommodation as a social response to it. This is not, of course, a matter of imposing on a structure whose meaning and purpose are clear a set of other meanings and purposes which are not. We cannot divorce the logic of secure accommodation from its social, political and legal uses, for these uses are themselves *part of* secure accommodation: secure accommodation is artefactual, the product of a discourse[1] containing a range of variably coherent and consensual beliefs about the social management of the deviant child. The wording, purpose and usage of law are, in this respect as in others, indistinguishable. Law is not the fount from which social acts spring, but is itself a social product, and by no means necessarily the most influential.

Hence we are dealing not with observable strata going down to a bedrock but with a perpetually and unpredictably shifting set of interrelations. Attempts at 'reform' by one actor in the process will provoke – as no doubt they were in turn provoked by – different and possibly conflicting actions by another. The social world differs from the natural scientist's laboratory in that, while the chemist's new compounds do not hit back, those of the social actor almost invariably do, and in ways which it is almost always difficult, and sometimes impossible, to predict, control or even manage.

In this chapter our main concern is with the temporal rather than spatial dimensions of secure accommodation, which is why our epigraph about the nascence of Dotheboys Hall is so relevant. Though our present arrangements are, by definition, contemporary, the problems with which they have to deal are not. Perhaps there never was a world in which family or community contained its difficulties harmoniously. If it contained them it did so, presumably, because it had fewer alternatives; if it did not, its failures may have gone unrecorded, for as the law did not intervene to help families with problems nor did it sanction the manner in which families controlled their children. Any problems which emerged in pre-industrial (and, the 'Domesday Book' notwithstanding, largely pre-statistical) Britain were private, unknown because unknowable, but by no means necessarily non-existent. Exporting children to notorious boarding schools with 'No Vacations' was, therefore, a product of and accommodation to a particular set of moral values and social opportunities. Whether, therefore, we are discussing early nineteenth-century Yorkshire boarding schools or late twentieth-century secure accommodation, we are analysing both continuities and discontinuities. Social actions are not simple responses to changes in the moral character of families – their methods of discipline, their capacity to instil religious beliefs, their child-raising practices – but central aspects of that character and, therefore, unlocked by reference not only to both family and state but also to the relations between them.

Whereas to the practitioner or administrator secure accommodation is a facility to be used as the law permits, to the social analyst it is a small corner of the social totality, a social product mediating the relations of state, family and child. A child causes or is the victim of a problem deemed to require a public solution of this socio-legal kind; but, it need hardly be stressed, both problem and solutions are the products of culture and history, not nature. Both the form and content of the child's deviance and the threshold and character of state intervention vary over time and place. While exclusion was once the predominant motif in child care, whether through institutions, migration, banishment or execution, it is now so residual that even exclusionary actions, of which it is hard to conceive of a better example than secure accommodation, demand not only justification but comprehension in the language and concepts of inclusion or rehabilitation. Part of the background to these historical mutations is the way in which popular definitions of the 'role of the state', the 'role of the family' and the 'nature of childhood' themselves have varied.

Even the common-sense division in western thought between 'I' and 'Society' is not God-given but the product of a particular historical conjunction (Althusser 1971; see also Ricoeur 1986: chs 7–9), a result of culture and history: Robinson Crusoe as *homo economicus* is a product of early mercantile capitalism infused with the Puritan ethic, not of a state of nature. Hence the very structures within which we define 'self', 'other', 'child', 'family', 'state' and 'society' are mutable. These categories, which seem to contemporary western eyes so natural, which divide us into units of individual, family, group, community and society, constitute that part of the discourse of our daily existence which linguistic theoreticians call the *langue* (Saussure 1974). To Saussure, language is far from being a mere representation of 'reality', but rather, by being both signifier and signified, a central feature of the social totality, the object as well as means of analysis. It comprises the *langue*, the system within which we not only speak and write but also construct meaning, and the *parole*, or the individual actualisation of the system. So while we may argue about 'family' as *parole* – whether or not, say, it incorporates grandchildren, nephews, stepchildren, cohabitees – we can only argue about family as *langue* if we allow for the existence of a structure which is 'not-family', so transforming the very meaning of those relationships – grandchildren, nephews and the rest – which emanate from it. The impossibility of doing so will be readily apparent, for these relationships are integral to the conceptual logic of our society and we cannot just 'step outside' them. There is, after all, no safe haven in which perception and analysis may unyoke themselves from those characteristics of contemporary society which so govern our perceptions of the world.[2]

This notion of the interdependence of words as component parts of a system is called 'synchronic solidarity':

> It is only when one understands this 'synchronic solidarity' that one really understands the meaning of an individual word. A visitor to western society might well learn that 'rape' means sex-by-force, yet never grasp the distinctive character that the word acquires in relation to such other words as 'love' and 'marriage'. Similarly, a visitor *from* western society might well learn that certain words in the language of an Indian tribe mean 'maternal uncle' and 'sister-in-law's brother', yet never grasp the interactions that lock all such family words into a system.
>
> (Harland 1987: 16)

State, family and childhood are interrelated, then, but in perpetually shifting ways. The notion that until recent times there was an institution called a 'private' family with absolute rights over its children and against the state is incorrect. When Ariès (of whom more later) observes,

> An analysis of iconography leads us to conclude that the concept of the family was unknown in the Middle Ages, that it originated in the fifteenth and sixteenth centuries, and that it reached its full expression in the seventeenth century.
>
> (Ariès 1962: 353)

he is referring to 'family' as a locus of permanence and security as we know it now: the medieval 'family' was an expedient, unstable structure, unrecognisable as the prototype of the conventional living unit of twentieth-century western society. Hence, to Duby, in medieval France:

> the family is the first refuge in which the threatened individual takes shelter when the authority of the State weakens. But as soon as political institutions afford him adequate guarantees, he shakes off the constraints of the family and the ties of blood are loosened. The history of lineage is a succession of contractions and relaxations whose rhythm follows the modifications of the political order.
>
> (Cited in Ariès 1962: 355)

To say, therefore, that the relation between family and state is variable over history is to speak not only of the relation, but of family and state themselves, for they, too, are ever-changing. Yet still a relation must exist, an accommodation between units of authority – individual, family and state. Often in the past these accommodations have centred on contemporary measures of social order: as the social functions of 'family' and 'line' in medieval France involved physical protection (through collective defence) and economic protection (through a necessary distribution of the inheritance), so did the main intervention of the courts in English family life prior to the mid-nineteenth century relate to the protection of those children who, as heirs to property, were made Wards in Chancery, subject to the jurisdiction of the court before that of the father or guardian (Pinchbeck and Hewitt 1973: 363). Though expressed in terms of economic rather than citizenship rights, the notion that it was the state's business to protect the child, albeit exclusively the child of property, was even then extant as an embodiment of the monarch's common law protective function of *parens patriae*.

This chapter proceeds as follows. First, we review a number of attempts by historians to identify continuities and discontinuities in relation to the family and childhood, and discover that there is an interesting lack of agreement among them on some central issues. We shall pause on these areas of disagreement, speculate briefly why they should leave us so perplexed, and proffer an alternative way forward. Secondly, we examine the work of Lorraine Fox Harding and her 'four perspectives' on child-care policy (Harding 1991). Though we are critical of the book, our main intent is to explore the *genre* rather than the example. Thirdly, to complement this critique we introduce briefly three concepts which, for our purposes, are indivisible. The interplay of *needs*, *rights* and *interests* is a crucial axis for our analysis of secure accommodation, for we argue that it is impossible to remove any one of them from secure accommodation without a disruption of understanding. There is no 'core' to secure accommodation; it exists rather as a set of shifting social actions and interactions, embracing any or all of our concepts, though in kaleidoscopically varying patterns depending on the particular 'case' in which it is interested. We shall conclude that to perceive secure accommodation as either undiluted altruism or oppressive incarceration cunningly disguised is to miss the essential point that precisely because it may be either, neither or both these things at different times, neither interpretation adequately encapsulates and expresses what secure accommodation 'is'.

To the reader who seeks a simple 'account' of contemporary secure accommodation, this approach may initially seem laboured. Straightforward accounts do exist elsewhere, however (Millham *et al.* 1978; Cawson and Martell 1979; Children's Legal Centre 1982; Blumenthal 1985; Bullock *et al.* 1990; and, from a practitioner's perspective, Hoghughi, M. 1984; Hoghughi, P. *et al.* n.d.), and we shall draw on them as we proceed. Our focus is different because our concern is not (at least not directly) normative; our intention is rather to paint a picture of what is done to difficult children today, what reasons are given for doing so, how the children themselves perceive their circumstances and what we believe these various actions signify.

SOME HISTORICAL ACCOUNTS

We do not offer a detailed history of child-care policy, for there exist already a literature on the child and the family in pre-industrial England, another offering a general overview of developments in child-care and juvenile justice and a third on secure accommodation itself. Our approach is rather to look with critical eye at what history claims to tell us, to enquire why things seem to have happened as they did and, from the rhythm of the various transformations chronicled by the historians – in political power, attitude, behaviour, theory – to grasp something of the place of secure accommodation and child care generally in the social totality.

Childhood itself has an interesting history. Neglected by conventional historians for many years – though see, of course, Rousseau (1762) and the idiosyncratic contribution of Boas (1966) – it became the subject of a monumental study by the French demographic historian Philippe Ariès, published in France in 1960 and in Britain, closely translated but with a significantly different title, two years later (Ariès 1960; 1962). Ariès's study was widely afforded seminal status, though, perhaps because it was less read than read about, a vulgarisation of its main thesis became part of received contemporary wisdom about childhood itself. Though Ariès decidedly did *not* say that there was in the past no concept (or 'idea') of childhood, he did claim, drawing on medieval iconography, that such a concept developed only gradually, from around the thirteenth century, that it shifted significantly between then and now, and that childhood was indeed very short. If there is a problem with Ariès's thesis it lies primarily in what, precisely he *means* by the 'idea' of childhood and in his confidence that the contemporary idea of childhood is so distinct from the contemporary idea of (even young) adulthood:

> In medieval society the idea of childhood did not exist; this is not to suggest that children were neglected, forsaken or despised. The idea of childhood is not to be confused with affection for children: it corresponds to an awareness of the particular nature of childhood, that particular nature which distinguishes the child from the adult, even the young adult. In medieval society this awareness was lacking.
>
> (Ariès 1962: 128)

As time moved on the child became first an object of 'coddling' based on the sheer sentimental joy experienced by its parents (in the sixteenth century) and then, under the influence of the moralists and churchmen of the seventeenth century, a small yet somewhat malevolent creature of God, in need of taming and training – a theme to which the nineteenth century was to return with renewed vigour. Ariès's thesis is that the 'natural' delight which parents took in their little child was destroyed by the influence of outside experts whose strictures on 'spoiling' and whose emphasis on discipline profoundly affected the patterns of family life (Ariès 1962: 132–3). Had it not been for these moralists:

> the child would have remained simply the *poupart* or *bambino*, the sweet, funny little creature with whom people played affectionately but with liberty, if not indeed with licence, and without any thought of morality or education. Once he had passed the age of five or seven, the child was immediately absorbed into the world of adults.
>
> (Ariès 1962: 329)

This trend involved the spontaneity of the bourgeois family (for the lower-class family for the most part escaped these pressures) being mediated from without, as parental affection came to be harnessed to the wider needs of the state to moralise the child. Alongside this, however, came a second phenomenon, also reflecting a new culture of bourgeois individualism, the privatisation of family life. Drawing both on changing iconography (interiors being rare in pre-seventeenth century European art) and on contemporary evidence of sexual openness with and among young children (also until the seventeenth century), Ariès argues that an increasing distance developed between the interiority of the family and the exteriority of the world. This 'distance' included a new emphasis on schooling which 'created' a childhood which no longer stopped pre-pubertally; in turn this division between the interior and exterior worlds met the needs of an emerging bourgeois culture for privacy and identity, but had its cost, especially for the nature of childhood:

> The old society concentrated the maximum number of ways of life into the minimum of space and accepted, if it did not impose, the bizarre juxtaposition of the most widely different classes. The new society, on the contrary, provided each way of life with a confined space in which it was understood that the dominant features should be respected, and that each person had to resemble a conventional model, an ideal type, and never depart from it under pain of excommunication.
>
> (Ariès 1962: 415)

So to Ariès the history of childhood is one of changing attitudes, beliefs and behaviours within the family and a changing relation between the family and those outside experts who, though then associated with the Church, would now be employed by the secular state. The results of these changes have been, first, the extension of the notion of bourgeois 'childhood' into the phase of sexual maturity (and so well beyond the common period of medieval marriage); secondly, a change in the meaning of 'childhood' by the creation of an image of the child in need of discipline and training; and, thirdly, the portrayal of family life as shifting from something 'public', characterised by *sociabilité* (Baldick's 'sociability' is a subtly misleading translation) to a 'private' domain of drab uniformity.

From all this we extract three themes and identify one point of departure from Ariès's phasic and substitutive analysis. First, we note that the 'extension' of childhood has been largely a bourgeois and aristocratic phenomenon; truncated childhood remained characteristic of the lower classes primarily because the interests of the exterior world in educating them were less strong. This difference re-emerges in the concept 'tutelage' (Donzelot 1980), for in the absence of the constraints which characterise bourgeois childhood lies a particular form of threat to social order. Whereas for the bourgeois child the pedagogic need is to cut the *cordon sanitaire* which its family has drawn round it, and to offer instead a '*protected liberation,* a freeing of children from vulgar fears and constraints', for the lower-class child the need is the opposite:

> it would be more exact to define the pedagogical model as that of *supervised freedom.* The problem in regard to the working-class child was not so much the weight of obsolescent constraints as excessive freedom – being left to the street – and the techniques employed consisted in limiting the freedom, in shepherding the child back to spaces where he could be more closely watched: the school or the family dwelling.
>
> (Donzelot 1980: 47)

This in turn, by stressing the interrelatedness of childhood, family and state, anticipates a crucial dimension of our own argument. The bourgeois family does for (or to) children what the state does *faut de mieux*, whereas the lower-class family, in permitting 'excessive' freedom, creates a potentially disruptive sense of autonomy in the immature or disaffected child. It is this that the state must control, whether by emulating the 'good' family or the 'firm' schoolmaster – respectively giving care and love to the 'neglected' child (for do we not perceive giving undue latitude to the unruly young as symptomatic of neglect?) and dispensing punishment to the miscreant who has abused this latitude.

The second theme is the involvement in this process of the 'experts'. Without doubt we see in the seventeenth-century moralists and pedagogues the state's creation and occupation of a prototypical conduit between the private domain of the family and the external world. Whether children were to study with the seventeenth-century clerics; whether following the Education Acts of the nineteenth century they were to be compulsorily educated; whether they were to have their working hours restricted by the

Factory Acts or their misconducts punished by the increasingly differentiated juvenile delinquency code; or whether they were to be protected against violence within the family (the Prevention of Cruelty to and Protection of Children Act was passed in 1889), they were gradually becoming citizens of the state, but with different rights and duties from those of adults, the differences accruing from their very status as children.

It would be a misunderstanding to regard the pre-twentieth-century child as simply the property of the father. The absence of a legal code or public statement on the 'rights' of the child should not be decontextualised: in all areas, not just those relating to children and families, the codification of civil and criminal law proceeded only slowly, and to conceive of the child as 'private property' because no law decreed otherwise would be to make a historical error. The law is not the engine which drives all social and micro-political relations; indeed, the wording of law can be almost incidental to the processes which occur, the actions people take, the strategies they develop. In the case of the bourgeois and aristocratic child there has been a notion of 'public interest' for many centuries, as there has been an economically driven common law interest in children who are heirs to property. While we know less of the state's interest in the children of the poor, the concept 'privacy' has changed over time, and prior to this century the notion of a poor family being 'private' in the sense that we understand the term today was inconceivable: a proletarian nuclear family claiming a 'right' to privacy is a product of late nineteenth- and twentieth-century liberal democracy, a fairly recent and, for all we know, short-lived mode of group living.

The third theme is that a crucial conjunction has occurred. The family as an institution has, from a long historical perspective, closed in more upon itself, become more private, at the very time that the developing social-welfare policies and legislation of the state have extended its remit into these private areas. The seventeenth century saw the beginning of these contrapuntal processes of the bourgeois family becoming more 'private' but the child becoming more 'public' – with the churchmen and moralists moving to a position of expertise and legitimacy in child rearing:

> In the moralists and pedagogues of the seventeenth century, we see that fondness for childhood and its special nature no longer found expression in amusement and 'coddling', but in psychological interest and moral solicitude. The child was no longer regarded as amusing or agreeable: 'Every man must be conscious of that insipidity of childhood which disgusts the sane mind; that coarseness of youth which finds pleasure in scarcely anything but material objects and which is only a very crude sketch of the man of thought.'
>
> (Ariès 1962: 131)

It is this conjunction which has contributed crucially to the relation of state, family and child today. An increasingly intrusive state facing an increasingly private family when childhood is associated with innocence and powerlessness is bound to be most poignant in the field of child abuse and child protection (Parton 1985; 1991; Harris 1990). In our field too, however, the relation, though ambiguous, is also crucial. The state steps in to socialise the unsocialised child, to transform into respectable citizens the products of other-than-respectable families. Secure accommodation is used when less intrusive forms of kindness and persuasion have failed. Crucially, however, secure accommodation is itself characterised by both kindness and persuasion as well as by sufficient coercion to compel acceptance of them. Only when we understand that this kindness is real, not a smokescreen for the imposition of control, however, can we begin to understand the nature of the power we are discussing. Power is not merely control masquerading as care, but both, not simultaneously but inextricably, as the flour and the egg, when beaten in the mixing bowl, yield a compound which, though comprising flour and egg, is recognisable as neither.

Finally, our point of departure from Ariès. Against his 'phasic' or *substitutive* view of childhood – the child becomes this in the sixteenth, that in the seventeenth century almost as though on a given day, month or year one set of beliefs was replaced by another – we offer a *cumulative* theory of cultural traces in order to explain that which is otherwise contradictory. The 'idea' of childhood does not make of the child a little angel to be coddled *or* a little devil to be tamed, a mini-adult, rational and calculating *or* a victim of passion, impulse and instinct, but any or all of them existing in dialectical relation to one another. Childhood is an accumulation of 'traces' which, if regarded separately, would indeed be contradictory but which cannot *be* regarded separately without missing the point: hence the argument which we shall later have with Lorraine Harding's 'value perspectives'. It is from this conceptual interrelatedness that the explanatory power of the experts derives, a point to which we return in Chapter 3. For the capacity to make strategic simplifications, to 'create' almost any image of the child from the rich data available in our cultural repertoire is immense.

Ariès's approach has been subjected to much critical attention (for convenient reviews see Pollock 1983: 28–32; Frost and Stein 1989: 12–14; Franklin 1986: ch. 1). Perhaps the most telling critique of Ariès's work is that of the empirical historian Linda Pollock (Pollock 1983). Pollock's use of primary sources (diaries, autobiographies and contemporary newspaper reports), from which she concludes that the nature and actions of family life have, over a long historical period, remained remarkably static, seeks to avoid what she regards as the methodological problems inherent in taking at face value such self-consciously normative public documents as tracts, sermons and the writings of experts.

Pollock's approach, however, is not without problems of its own, for she comes close to regarding her primary sources as yielding data which have an objectivity, or at least reliability, which seems to us impossible. Neither the autobiography nor the newspaper account lacks a subtext, neither can be unyoked from its own socio-cultural context, and for the historian to avoid texts containing overt authorial didacticism is not to achieve objectivity but to uncover a different, possibly more subtle, mode of representation. As with Ariès's changing concept 'family', the signifiers may stay the same but what is signified may not. The (auto)biographer creates a rationale for selection on the basis of values, beliefs and assumptions which make individual and cultural sense. The outcome is inevitably variable, as the most cursory consideration of different biographies respectively lauding and vilifying the same 'subject' makes plain. Foucault's biographer, Didier Eribon, engaging in what he acknowledges to be the paradoxical activity of writing a biography of a subject who has decisively repudiated the concept 'author-ity', discusses this point more fully: '*Il peut sembler paradoxal d'écrire une biographie de Michel Foucault. N'avait-il pas à plusieurs reprises récusé la notion d'auteur, bannissant par conséquent la possibilité même d'une étude biographique?*' (Eribon 1991: 11). Other problems, though regarded by Eribon as relating especially to his particular subject, are probably universal for the biographer: not only Foucault but all subjects are multi-faceted; none, surely, has a simple 'core' through to which to penetrate:

> *Mais, concernant Foucault, il y avait des difficultés particulières. Il était un personnage complexe et multiple. 'Il portait des masques, et il en changeait toujours', disait de lui Dumézil, qui le connaissait mieux de quiconque. Je n'ai pas cherché à révéler 'la' verité de Foucault; sous le masque, il y a toujours un masque, et je ne pense pas qu'il y ait une vérité de la personnalité qu'il serait possible de retrouver sous des déguisements successifs. Il y a plusieurs Foucault? Mille Foucault, comme disait Dumézil? Oui, sans doute. Je les ai présentés tels qu'ils me sont apparus.*
>
> (Eribon 1991: 13)

In the case of the diary we encounter the problem that the document, though conventionally perceived as private, embodies a curious notion of privacy, for its existence paradoxically threatens or destroys the very privacy of its contents. We do not know why or for whom the diarist is 'really' writing, what story of the self is being created; but to assume the story is 'objective' cannot be correct, for as with Foucault, '*sous le masque, il y a toujours un masque*'. At one level it is common for diarists to seek, consciously or not, a degree of narrative consistency in their work. Leonard Woolf, defending his own heavy editing of his wife's diary, makes the point perfectly:

> At the best and even unexpurgated, diaries give a distorted portrait of the writer, because, as Virginia Woolf herself remarks somewhere in these diaries, one gets into the habit of recording one particular kind of mood – irritation or misery, say – and of not writing one's diary when one is feeling the opposite. The portrait is therefore from the start unbalanced.
> (Woolf 1953: vii–viii)

More theoretically, all communications tell us only what they tell us, not what 'was' but what was selected by the writer; a diary is a narrative and tells us what the narrator wished to communicate, not the *histoire* or what 'really happened' (Genette 1980). Contrary both to conventional western rationalist discourse and to the central quest of Husserl's and Schutz's phenomenology (Husserl 1970; Schutz 1972), the idea that an unmediated relation between reader and signified 'reality' does or can exist must be regarded with circumspection (any such idea is, indeed, effectively demolished by Eagleton 1983: 55–66). Similar circumspection must be afforded Pollock's quest for objectivity. Her biographies, newspapers and diaries are of course informative, indeed loquacious, but then so are moral tracts and 'scientific' studies, and all of them in the same way: they tell us, reliably, much about the representational mode, but we cannot rely on them for an objective account of the events themselves.

If the problem Pollock is trying to solve were evidential, involving the exposure and elimination of the lie, her impeccable cross-checking and analysis of primary sources would suffice. If, though, the problem involves comprehending the significations of 'words' from a different time and place and translating them into terms comprehensible to the late-twentieth-century reader, the method is fallible, as our epigraph about Flaubert's gianthood is intended to demonstrate. For example, Pollock shows us that parents were not 'cruel' and that they 'loved' their children much as we supposedly do today. Both cruelty and love, however, are, at least in western Judaeo-Christian cultures, universal moral attributes of 'bad' and 'good' respectively, and we should expect them, therefore, to feature in historical documents about how people lived. Operationally, however, both concepts are mutable, and it does not quite work to conclude from the fact that we share a Judaeo-Christian culture with our distant ancestors that our forms of behaviour have remained static over time. To any Christian society a 'cruel' parent must be abnormal because no such society can logically conceive of cruelty as normal. It is, however, perfectly possible for the outside observer from a different time or place to pass judgement on the merits of what was accepted or not in a different place or at a different time in terms of, say, disciplining, education, play and religious instruction.

Pollock, like other critics of Ariès, also has a tendency to regard the supposed absence of a concept of childhood as meaning simply that the child was regarded as a small adult without special needs, and it is this apparent belief which she challenges. This notion of conceptless childhood has come to be associated, therefore, with a form of cruelty based on the assumption that a child is more simply rational than we currently believe to be the case, even though Ariès himself distinguishes the idea of childhood from the question of kindness to children. Other writers do not make this distinction, however, and Pollock, on the basis of newspaper reports of the trials of child abusers, mounts a telling criticism of the undoubtedly incorrect inferences of two British social historians (Pinchbeck and Hewitt 1969, 1973):

> Pinchbeck & Hewitt refer to the case of one woman who put out the eyes of a child in her care in order that the child might then earn money by begging. They claim that it was only because the woman was employed by the parish to look after children that her cruelty was prosecuted and that, if the woman had been the child's mother, no one would have bothered to intervene because it was accepted that parents could treat their offspring as they pleased. Thus they infer from one particular case the attitude of the whole of 18th- and 19th-century society to children.
>
> (Pollock 1983: 91–2)

Pinchbeck and Hewitt's relatively simple position is not, however, that of Ariès, to whom the undoubted cruelties of the nineteenth century were if anything a 'retrogression' (Ariès 1962: 336) to medieval society. Contrast this too with the view of Lloyd deMause (and a weaker historical imagination it would be hard to imagine) that: 'The further back in history one goes, the lower the level of child care, and the more likely children are to be killed, abandoned, beaten, terrorized, and sexually abused' (deMause 1976: 1). To Ariès it was, as we have seen, the lower class which had withstood the attacks on freedom by education experienced by the bourgeois family:

> Child labour retained this characteristic of medieval society: the precocity of the entry into adult life. The whole complexion of life was changed by the differences in the educational treatment of the middle-class and the lower-class child.
>
> (Ariès 1962: 336)

If anything, Pollock's scrupulous study of contemporary sources implies a theory not of change but of stasis in child rearing: to Pollock, once one gets behind the public statements of what is 'good' or 'bad' practice and comes closer to the ways in which parents actually behaved (about which she claims other historical methods tell us little) and the attitudes and beliefs they held, '[m]any parental attitudes to children discovered from the primary sources turn up again in 20th-century parents' (Pollock 1983: 141). Parents mourned the deaths of children much as they do now, their responses to children's illnesses were also more similar to than different from our own, as were their concerns about education and welfare. Pollock does not, however, explain, or even make explicit, any *theory* of stasis, taking it as a social fact yielding only to her methodology of studying private documents and newspaper reports:

> It is vital to understand why most parents do not and did not subject their children to the level of unremitting severity and cruelty which has been claimed . . . . Hutchinson related the tale of an acquaintance who replied to some advice on child-rearing with 'that's no use to me. If he was your son so would I jolly well know what to do with him. The trouble is he's mine!' . . . parents are prepared to tolerate most of what would be considered wayward behaviour by others from their own children.
>
> (Pollock 1983: 201)

In other words, there is a gap between public statement and private reality. Public statements come and go but family love continues in subterranean form coming from – we know not where, for Pollock, though an excellent empirical historian, is no social theorist.

'PERSPECTIVES' ON CHILD-CARE POLICY: A CRITIQUE

The apparently simple question of the relations of family, child and state is, therefore, permeated by complexity and obscurity, containing a knowledge vacuum which it is often difficult to resist filling with easy but possibly incorrect answers. It is also tempting, and doubtless ultimately desirable, to attempt to classify these relations, but there are pitfalls for the unwary in so doing. In this section we consider critically one attempt, by Lorraine Harding, to develop a typology of the relations between the state and the family in child care. She regards these relations as reflecting four 'value perspectives' – *laissez-faire* and patriarchy; state paternalism and child protection; the modern defence of the birth family and parents' rights; and children's rights and child liberation (Harding 1991).

Harding devotes a long chapter to each of these 'value perspectives', concluding with two much shorter and less satisfactory chapters, 'Convergences and divergences' and 'Law, policy and practice: an uneasy synthesis'. While the main strengths of the book lie in the sections which, in reviewing established child-care writings in relation to her perspectives provide some excellent references, our interest is primarily in the issues with which she is attempting to deal in the later chapters. It is therefore on these that we shall concentrate.

Even in those chapters which represent the core of the book, however, the argument is not seamless. The seams show in two main ways. First, the perspectives are themselves expressed dualistically – *laissez-faire* and patriarchy, state paternalism and child protection, the modern defence of the birth family and parents' rights, children's rights and child liberation – and in spite of Harding's defence of these associations there is not invariably an obvious or necessary relation between the 'twin' dimensions of each.

Secondly, in those sections where she assigns authors to different camps we see clearly that it does not quite work. So the same authors appear in multiple camps: Allison Morris and her colleagues (Morris *et al.* 1980) are associated with *laissez-faire* and patriarchy *and* with children's rights and children's liberation (Harding 1991: 23); Robert Dingwall and his colleagues (Dingwall *et al.* 1983) may be surprised to find themselves placed in the state paternalism and child protection camp given that they are described as critical of 'heavy-handed paternalism' (Harding 1991: 64); and Michael Freeman (1983), who appears as a 'moderate' member of his camp – in this case 'children's rights and child liberation' – having launched a strong attack on some children's liberationists describes *himself* as a liberal paternalist. And since Harding notes that some of Freeman's criticisms of the response to child abuse resemble those of Robert Holman, whom she places in the 'defence of the birth family/parents' rights' camp (Harding 1991: 175), Freeman appears to lack a presence in only one of the four available camps.

Even in its own terms, therefore, there exist some serious problems with the typology. *Perspectives in Child Care Policy* is a good teaching book but weak as social theory. Our main interest, however, is less in the limitations of the analysis itself than in those of the genre of which it is a part. Indeed, it may be that the former largely result from the latter, which would explain why Harding encountered such evident difficulty in bringing the book to a conclusion.

In the first of the two concluding chapters, 'Convergences and divergences', Harding begins by acknowledging the very problems with her typology to which we have already referred: classifying authors, she admits, 'has not been entirely successful' (Harding 1991: 200). She then devotes four rather awkward pages to describing some very generalised convergences between some or all of her positions and ten rather more confident ones to analysing the divergences which appear as soon as we scratch the surface and start asking what concepts like 'best interests' and 'rights' actually mean. The final chapter, 'Law, policy and practice: an uneasy synthesis', struggles hard to relate her approach to the messy reality of 1980s child-care policies. It is less a sophisticated analysis than a selection of random thoughts from *Social Trends*, and it does not lead to a synthesis, however uneasy:

> Other factors in late post-War society which may be mentioned include smaller families, changes in sexual mores, changing gender roles and the influence of feminism, increasing demands on the 'middle' generations by the elderly, the demands from vulnerable and dependent groups discharged from hospital . . . . The relationship of all these variables to child care problems and the need for state intervention is complex, not clearcut; but the general point is that child care problems and the response to them do not arise in a social vacuum.
>
> (Harding 1991: 224)

She concludes by pondering whether the 1980s involved dealing with what she regards as the messy business of 'conflict' or the rational process of 'balance', hinting optimistically that the latter may be the case. There are, however, two main problems with this approach. The first, and less radical, is how best to conceptualise the relations among the different perspectives; we shall show that linguistic and conceptual confusion prevent Harding from developing her argument as she might. The second is whether it is theoretically correct (as well as heuristically convenient) to speak of perspectives in the first place.

First, the relation among the 'perspectives' is unclear. Though Harding herself is usually cheerfully eclectic, her thesis seems to be that the more 'coherent' (in her terms) the policy is, the better it will be. In almost any area of public policy, however, as Harding rightly observes, there exist conflicting objectives, perspectives and interests, and it is the business of policy makers and practitioners to 'balance' them (though 'accommodate' is, for reasons we shall later explain, a better word).

At this point Harding distinguishes 'balance' and 'conflict' (Harding 1991: 230–1). This, however, is clearly a confusion, for it is precisely conflicting objectives which have to be balanced. Harding requires a further explanatory concept, 'contradiction', to escape this muddle, for it is in relation to contradictory, not conflicting, objectives that 'balance' is impossible (Harris 1990: 337). Contradiction signifies a situation in which the pursuit of a given objective renders the pursuit of a given other objective a logical impossibility; conflict is one in which the pursuit of two objectives, though technically difficult, is not impossible. So walking towards and away from a stationary object at the same time would be a contradiction; simultaneously knitting and watching television would not.

If, therefore, to take an example from Harding, it were the case that 'more power for social workers in relation to children does mean that parents lose some of their rights' (Harding 1991: 230), to seek to increase the powers of social workers *and* the rights of parents would indeed be a contradictory objective. In such a situation the powers of the one and the rights of the other would exist in hydraulic relation, as in the distribution of a finite amount of water between two glasses: the more water we put in one glass the less is left to go in the other.

In the world of social policy, however, this analogy does not hold: not only is the *quantity* of power variable (whereas that of the water is constant) but also it is possible simultaneously to increase powers *and* to circumscribe the circumstances in which they may be exercised (see also Benton 1982). This is precisely the thrust of the changes in sentencing policy of the 1980s and early 1990s. We are not, therefore, dealing with contradiction, for one can simultaneously strengthen the powers of A *and* the rights of B against A's misuse of them.

There is also a problem with the concept 'balance'. 'Balance' implies the measured creation or recognition of a situation in which equal weights of two commodities exist on an actual or metaphorical pair of scales. Hence the appropriateness of the scales metaphor to the idea of a system of retributive justice: the 'gravity' (the very word means heaviness) of the crime must be balanced by the 'weight' of punishment. In child-care policy, however, we are not dealing with different commodities 'balanced' thus but with human judgements about how a range of factors should contribute to a decision which is, literally, in imbalance, affording precedence to one set of values over another. Thus the issue is not one of precise measurement but of a process which draws its 'meaning' from the social, not the quantitative, world. Though we do not seek to make heavy weather of this point, tropes like metaphor and metonymy create as well as convey meanings (Wicker 1975: *passim*), and we do not wish to encourage a metaphor of 'scales' which implies either the elimination or minimisation of human choice, or that a form of pure reason can emerge from 'balance'. Hence our preference for 'accommodation'.

In Harding's terms, therefore, different relations may exist between the perspectives. Her analysis is insufficiently precise or sophisticated to form the basis of a typology of the various possible combinations, nor is her reasoning in political philosophy sufficiently acute to lead her to prescribe some combinations and proscribe others. Though she refers briefly and intermittently to the Children Act 1989, part of the purpose of which is precisely the creation of new accommodations among state, family and child (Parton 1991), she offers little that is new about, for example, the concept 'responsibility' (Eekelaar 1991) or the presumption of no court order.

She fails also to identify any contradictory combinations of perspectives, and this leads us directly on to our second, more fundamental, problem, which stems from a difficulty to which we have already drawn attention. Just as few authors cited fit comfortably into one and only one perspective, so presumably would very few of us reject any one, two or three of the perspectives in favour of the fourth. Hence Harding's perspectives are not true 'alternatives' so much as culturally conventional (and therefore comprehensible) ways of describing and dividing a social totality. To most of us there is merit in all four, and, this being so, their typological utility is somewhat limited. Because they emerge from our cultural and intellectual reservoir of social, political and moral philosophy they constitute a familiar framework within which to approach difficult choices, but they cannot easily guide those choices themselves. To believe in privacy *and* protection of the vulnerable, in sympathy *and* punishment, is not to be logically or morally inconsistent as the location of these commitments in different perspectives would imply (else why have the perspectives at all?) but to expose the perspectives themselves as potentially misleading. The process of 'analysis', therefore, even as part of a prolonged intellectual exegesis designed to conclude in 'synthesis', does not explicate 'reality' but creates or confirms a certain conventional and therefore comprehensible ordering of ideas. In the practical world of policy making we still have to accommodate these perspectives in particular 'cases'. As Harding herself notes, in a curiously vague passage which both reminds us that the perspectives *qua* perspectives are unreal, non-existent even, and that to create them can confuse more than it clarifies:

> While each perspective has a degree of internal coherence, and while each may be identified as influential in actual policy and practice at different times and in different places, the 'real world' of such policy and practice, it is argued, always represents an uneasy and incoherent synthesis [*sic*] of views. That is, the perspectives are not found in practice in anything like their pure forms, notwithstanding the broad prominence of particular perspectives at times. Many factors influence the movements in *actual* policies. Among these, nevertheless, are swings in professional and pressure group thinking which may correspond to the perspectives which have been outlined.
>
> (Harding 1991: 217)

Though the process of ideal type analysis, of which Harding's book is an example, is an established method of western scientific enquiry which can indeed identify the strands in a complex set of interrelations and lead to a synthesis, it can also deceive us into believing that the strands exist as isolated phenomena, not as indissoluble parts of a shifting and restless whole. When the analysis patently fails to end in synthesis it can illumine neither form nor content, the source or nature of human action in the social world. It is a unidimensional account of a multi-faceted phenomenon, necessary perhaps but insufficient to engage with the linguistic, definitional, conceptual and operational complexities of state, family and child, and seriously misleading if we apply it to the study of secure accommodation.

RIGHTS, NEEDS AND INTERESTS: AMBIGUITY IN ACTION

> But people seldom act from one motive alone; if they do they are said to be obsessed.
>
> (Muriel Spark 1988: 43)

If the various dimensions comprising the totality of secure accommodation are neither to be analytically dissected nor simply 'balanced', and if we are to deny sovereignty to any one of them on the ground that the interrelation is greater than the sum of the parts, how are we to proceed, and how in particular to comprehend the workings of secure accommodation?

To understand how exigencies are appreciated in the light of secure accommodation, how decisions are reached to apply for authorisations and how resources, including available concepts, are used to respond to the exigencies, we must consider in some detail the main actors. This we shall do later in the book, but as we do so, turning to the interaction of the social workers and the young people, we shall not be entering a different world from the one we are presently studying: we shall still be in that world as constituted. The considerations workers entertain, the ways in which secure accommodation is envisaged by social workers and young people, the decisions to apply for an authorisation or to grant it are enacted in an arena that has now become fully politized, a part of the public argument of a polity.

Our historical account has shown that the provision of security was originally exclusively a matter of changed routine of a professional or technical interest, the objective being the maintenance of a system. The provision was of little interest to those outside the system, and problems could be solved through internal change within the system. Different audiences have become involved over the years, and different issues of security have been defined by interest groups, as a secure system has been at least partly differentiated from the care system in which 'security' had its unremarked origins. 'Security' has attracted the close attention of a department of state, an influential child-rights lobby and indeed the general public.

This widening of audience has increased the conceptual turbulence as different publics struggle to assert their understanding. So, in Hardingesque manner, champions emerge in support of the sovereignty of particular concepts to envisage the provision and to repudiate its use: claiming, for instance, that secure accommodation is not ambiguous but a prison; that the practice of social work in respect of secure accommodation should be described exclusively in terms of 'securing' the rights of young people. As bureaucrats, professionals and pressure groups struggle to make secure accommodation intelligible they have no choice but to use notions – such as rights, needs and interests – which are contested, or at least unsettled, in the wider society. Interest groups see no necessity for any close attention to conceptual complexity, the unravelling of which is often dismissed as academic indulgence or even self-interest. However, as the topic of secure accommodation has entered the rhetoric of a number of publics, so have the use and usage of the available notions of rights, needs and interests permeated a domain which can no longer be addressed exclusively in professional or administrative terms. Our consideration of the general use of these ideas as part of the process of examining particular attempts to render secure accommodation intelligible is no academic mystery tour: they are key elements in the main action.

The main concepts used to make the provision of secure accommodation intelligible – *rights, needs, interests* – have a long history and a voluminous and controversial literature. Our necessarily brief consideration would be merely self-defeating were it not that we have two relatively modest objectives: to illustrate the contested nature of each of the concepts and also the extent to which they are interrelated. The range of differences in use has practical consequences, and understanding the interrelationship of the three concepts provides the foundation for good practice in the light and vicinity of secure accommodation.

We might consider, when we come to examine their cases, that some at least of the young people in secure accommodation are in great *need*. Need is an idea that has figured centrally in social welfare discussion: so services should be distributed according to measured needs, people understood in terms of common human needs. Yet 'needs' has no generally agreed place in welfare discourse. For some the notion is akin to that of phlogiston in an earlier age, whilst others see 'need' as playing an essential part in the definition of the main area of social policy study. Some believe that 'needs' constitutes an unnecessarily complicated way of referring to wishes or at least those wishes that can be marshalled into demands. Others detect something sinister in the complication:

An emphasis upon needs as opposed to wants cannot but appeal to those

> who would like to see themselves as experts qualified both to determine what the needs of others are, and to prescribe and enforce the means appropriate to the satisfaction of those needs.
>
> (Flew 1981: 117)

Welfare experts, whose confidence has, as we have seen, been undermined, may prefer to attend to what people want rather than become involved in making judgements about what people, especially young people, need. We shall see this tendency in action in Chapters 4 and 5 in particular, and it is increased the more it is appreciated that 'the concept of need is . . . one of the most elusive and open-ended to be found in the arena of political discourse' (Campbell 1983: 133).

It is possible, however, to reduce the elusiveness and the contradiction in interpretation. Garrett Thomson, for example, considers the range of use of the concept by posing three major questions: is the notion of need normative in itself or do we have to establish separately that what people can be said to need ought to be supplied? Does 'need' always entail a lack of some kind? Should we see 'needs' as offering some kind of explanation of behaviour through the descriptions of states of tension which will persist until relieved, or have 'needs' no part to play in the explanation of human conduct (Thomson 1987)?

Thomson resolves these dilemmas by making use of the simple but crucial distinction between two main uses of the idea of needs, the *instrumental* and the *normative* (Thomson 1987: 7–9). Griffin has pointed to the importance of distinguishing needs arising from the ends we happen to have chosen and needs we all have because we are human (Griffin 1986). The first indicates a certain relation of necessity and carries no justificatory weight, as in the phrase quoted by Thomson – in order to conduct electricity an element 'needs' a free election – or, in the terminology of this book, a person 'needs' to be in 'secure accommodation' to be the subject of any treatment or attention at all.

The second use is normative – the young person is in need of security – and constitutes a prima facie claim that what is 'needed' cannot be dispensed with and cannot be forgone without serious harm. Harm, however, is a problematic concept, applicable not only to the experiences of 'harmed' individuals, but affecting also the social fabric which is itself 'integral to our personhood' (Kleinig 1978: 36). For Thomson, harm is no temporary misfortune but a degeneration in the quality of life which must continue until we have that which we need (Thomson 1987: ch. III). Talk of 'needs' in the non-instrumental sense helps us discern what ought to be done in the name of self-interest, either in our own case or in that of others. This understanding of fundamental need seems very close to Campbell's 'welfare principle' or the prescription that 'each person ought to receive or be left in possession of that which is necessary to meet his or her basic, course-of-life needs' (Campbell 1983: 134).

Thomson's general treatment of needs is relevant to our present argument in two ways. First, the distinction between instrumental and fundamental needs disarms those who would divorce 'needs' from welfare discourse, since such arguments rely on only one meaning of the notion. It could also assist those who require an elaborated notion in order to direct attention 'from needs to discourses about needs, from the distribution of need satisfaction to "the politics of need interpretation"' (Fraser 1989: 292). Fraser's argument would have been considerably strengthened if she had not relied exclusively on an instrumental interpretation of 'needs'. After all, a need of shelter in order to live is scarcely a paradigmatic illustration of the instrumental use of 'needs'.

Similarly, the distinction between fundamental and instrumental need constitutes the ground for the useful differentiation made by Penz (1986) between condition needs and assistance needs. The former refer to a lack in a person's situation and the latter to what is required as a response to a condition. Thomson's discussion also points to the interrelatedness of talk about needs, what people want and what is in their interests.

Interests, our second concept, are distinct from wants or preferences (Benton 1982); they cannot simply be read off what we discover or know someone wants. We shall encounter a concrete example of this distinction in Chapter 4, when we discover the concern experienced by social workers that there are children who actually *want* to go into secure accommodation. To Benton, any notion of interests is indispensably evaluative and accordingly essentially contested. If we want to assert the presence of 'interests', no special place can be given to self-ascription as distinct from other-ascription. The assessment of interests, either one's own or those of others, involves two operations: the evaluation of evidence and taking into account various considerations. Benton suggests that relevant evidence will include information about circumstances, present and future, personal and social identity, preferences and ambitions of the subject; whilst considerations will include the application of moral, prudential and/or political standards and principles to the circumstances, preferences and ambitions.

In so far as the ascription of interests rests on considerations, Benton argues, they are contestable but not demonstrably true or false; in so far as they are based on evidence, they are both contestable and in principle demonstrably true or false. Finally, there are intimate conceptual links between interests and personal and social identities. Benton suggests that in so far as an individual is socially constituted as a member of a family, anything that has a bearing on the well-being of other family members also has a bearing on the interests of that person:

> These features of the concept of 'interests' fit it to play a multiplicity of roles in a variety of discourses and related social practices in which identities are formed and transformed, in which conflicts of loyalty are resolved, in which specific courses of action are urged or opposed and in which exercises of power are legitimated.
>
> (Benton 1982: 30)

The third of the notions we are considering, that of *rights*, also is subject to a range of uses. As Jones commented in a review of recent writing on the subject, there is little concerning rights that is not disputed (Jones 1989; see also Spicker 1988: ch. V). We as a society are in dispute about what we actually mean when we say, as we frequently do, that it is a 'right' that, for instance, children should play. What kind of a claim is this, and against what or whom should it be pressed? Is rights-talk a homogeneous language, so that we are in the perspective of a single genus, though particular species may be identified? Here we should attend to the kind of clarification advanced by theoretical jurists such as Hohfeld, that 'rights' can be classified as of a kind: as liberties, claims, immunities and powers (Hohfeld 1923; Timms 1986 applies this classification to the social work concept of self-determination). Though some argue that Hohfeld's classification system falls short of homogeneity, or that only claims may properly be treated as rights:

> we should not confuse the typical occasion for invoking a right with its meaning. At any particular time I have the right to do (am 'at liberty' to do) the indefinitely many things I am not prohibited from doing, even though I may not even think about them, be challenged or make claims about them.
>
> (Jones 1989: 69)

Other controversies concerning the basis and the content of rights are intensified when attention is focused on those rights that are termed 'natural' or 'human' (for critical discussions of Cranston's restrictive view of human rights, see Plant *et al.* 1980; Spicker 1988). Campbell argues this from a socialist perspective (Campbell 1983), while Gewirth justifies human rights to freedom and to well-being through depicting the necessary conditions of human action: a person

> has rights to freedom and well-being because these goods are due to him from within his own standpoint as a prospective purposive agent, since

> he needs these goods in order to act either at all or with the general possibility of success.
>
> (Gewirth 1982: 50)

The objective of this brief incursion into rather dense conceptual thickets has primarily been to establish the contested and the connected nature of talk about needs, interests and rights and to stress the necessity of accommodating all of them, for all are inextricable aspects of the complex relation of family, state and child. Fraser is of the view that 'this peculiar juxtaposition of a discourse about needs with discourses about rights and interests is one of the distinctive marks of late-capitalist political culture' (1989: 292). Our discussion suggests that the relationship between these notions is other than peculiar and more than one of simple juxtaposition, more than one of 'balance', a set of arrangements with a logic which is integrated in the sense that any one part of it derives its 'meaning' and purpose from one or more of the other parts.

TOWARDS A CONCLUSION

> And what about the canonisation of certain critical theorists as opposed to others? Arguments objecting to the canonisation of Shakespeare and to the tyranny of 'author-ity' often contain appeals to the critical authority of surnames intoned like those of saints: instead of, say, 'just Marlowe' we have 'just Lacan', or 'Derrida' or 'Foucault'. So what else is new?
>
> (Hawkins 1990: 108)

Perspectives such as Harding's do not act as *ante hoc* referents for the social actor. When faced with a difficulty we do not have conscious resort to a piece of moral or political philosophy by means of which to resolve it. When we hear a child scream we do not remind ourselves that we are (say) child liberationists not paternalists and programme our response accordingly. The forms of value or knowledge which people bring to bear in their professional activities are less likely to be of this abstract kind than strategic, a version of the skills used to solve any other problem based on what is, in a particular if all-embracing, sense 'experience' (Oakeshott 1933).

Of course these skills must be presented, and are indeed likely to be understood, in a particular way, for the 'value perspectives' represent the public 'discourse' of liberal professionalism and as such have a reality of their own. The fact that the act does not come from the idea (as though the act could be dependent on the idea for its fruition), does not mean that it is independent of it, as though the idea were mere *post hoc* justification. The idea makes sense of and gives logic and integrity to the act while also providing the frame of reference within which the act can be socially, intellectually and morally grasped. The 'explanation' of the act is neither 'true' nor 'false' but a product of the same social, cultural and intellectual milieu, a part of the act itself. This is why it is simultaneously possible for Harding to *place* her writers within the discourse of four perspectives and impossible for her to *encapsulate* them in any one of the four. The perspectives represent a shared language, a representation of reality but not reality itself.

If, though, the issue is not one of the idea leading to the act, nor is it, conversely, one of deception, as though a 'real' reason were being conspiratorially denied, with false altruism attached to an act of cynical self-interest. To make such a claim would be to confuse 'presentation' with 'deception'. Deception involves saying that which the sayer knows to be false with the intention of misleading – that one did not kill one's victim, beat one's wife, steal the petty cash when one knows one did. Presentation is a more complex activity, acknowledging that almost any social 'fact' has potentially multiple interpretations. To offer one interpretation in a particular setting involves a process of selection which may (of course) be strategic and self-interested, but which may also seek to create consonance among explanation, context and purpose. So the explanation, when 'presented' in any form of communication, whether for formal purposes such as office records or forensic evidence or for informal purposes such as tea-room chat, renders the action comprehensible by locating it within the shared and acceptable discourse of speaker and listener, or writer and reader. The same act may, therefore, be 'explained' in moral or professional terms for the records or the court; or, in the world of the tea room, cynically or commonsensically. While each of these 'explanations' changes the 'meaning' of the act itself, to give a 'total' explanation of any multi-faceted act would be a practical and conceptual impossibility, and to present it differently in different contexts is not necessarily to deceive.[3]

Our concern is to step outside of what is technically termed 'logocentrism' by allowing that no single, fundamental, essential 'reason' for an act may exist, but rather a multiplicity of 'reasons' seldom clear even to the actor. This takes us well beyond the Harding notion of 'value perspectives'. 'Logocentrism' is the term coined by Jacques Derrida in part to explain the comforting but false idea that there is a 'reality', a 'centre' to everything (Derrida 1976; see also Selden 1985: 88, and, for an accessible discussion of Derrida's critique of western thought, Boyne 1990: ch. 4 and *passim*). The neologism refers to one of the earliest pieces of logocentrism, 'In the beginning was the Word' – the concept *logos* carrying, as the Biblical context makes clear, a far greater concentration of power and spirit than its much diluted English formulation (Derrida 1976: 98). It is as logocentric to argue cynically that the 'centre' is deceit – fine words concealing foul deeds – as it is to argue naïvely that the altruistic value should be the core of the matter. To allow simultaneously for both truth and deceit is to avoid the logocentric fallacy and to approach a new and multi-faceted version of 'reality'. If we miss this point we shall miss some of the major characteristics both of secure accommodation and of the youngsters it contains.

In the case of secure accommodation there are two distinct forms of logocentric discourse. The first is that secure accommodation is benign, caring, therapeutic, designed above all to meet the best interests of the child who is forever running away from problems. Skilled and caring staff will provide the youngster with a 'secure' framework within which greater confidence and maturity can be gained. The second form, encapsulated in the phrase 'locking up children', is that all this is a fraudulent attempt to make us forget that secure accommodation is a form of imprisonment of the young, but without the safeguards which attend other custodial provisions. It is thus a form of insidious state power designed less to enhance the well-being of the child than to control the deviant and provide job opportunities for the professionals.

In the first of these analyses, secure accommodation is perceived naïvely, in the second, cynically, so that *naïveté* and cynicism are, respectively, at the 'heart' of the enterprise. If, though, we can allow that secure accommodation is both these things simultaneously, we not only avoid a crude and culture-bound 'either–or' squabble about secure accommodation, but more fundamentally we can perceive something of the true nature of power. The kindness and concern are genuine – one needs only to speak to the professionals and magistrates concerned to appreciate that – yet still the doors are locked and the children forced to stay. And it is precisely in this integration of kindness and control that we perceive the totality of the power of secure accommodation.

Roland Barthes provides one of the best-known examples of this point, using the concept 'myth' to explicate the relation between form and content. Describing a poster which shows a black soldier proudly saluting the French national flag he ponders the 'meaning and the form' of this particular 'myth'. To receive the poster naïvely is to regard the soldier as a *symbol* for French imperiality, a statement about unity, honour, fidelity; to take it as a deception is to regard the soldier as an *alibi* for French imperiality, a crude and calculated political piece of propaganda; but

> if I focus on the mythical signifier as on an inextricable whole made of meaning and form, I receive an ambiguous signification: I respond to the constituting mechanism of myth, to its own dynamics, I become a reader of myths. The saluting Negro is no longer an example or a symbol, still

> less an alibi: he is the very *presence* of French imperiality. . . . If the reader does not see French imperiality in the saluting Negro, it was not worth weighting the latter with it; and if he sees it, the myth is nothing more than a political proposition, honestly expressed.
>
> (Barthes 1973: 139–40)

None of which is to deny that propaganda exists: indeed it is self-evidently ubiquitous. Rather, it is to break any simple equation between 'propaganda' and falsehood, for the simplicity of such a formulation would clearly, except so far as the simple-minded were concerned, emasculate the propaganda itself: it would leave unanswered the question of how people could 'believe' (accept as 'true') that which they 'knew' to be propaganda (and therefore 'false'). 'Propaganda', however, as a moment's consideration of the influence of the advertisement on human purchasing behaviour reminds us, is itself conceptually problematic: meaning and form coexist as much in the mind of the recipient as in the purpose of the communicator; we can seldom escape the power of the myth:

> In a single day, how many really non-signifying fields do we cross? Very few, sometimes none. Here I am, before the sea; it is true that it bears no message. But on the beach, what material for semiology! Flags, slogans, signals, sign-boards, clothes, suntan even, which are so many messages to me.
>
> (Barthes 1973: 121)

In this sense, to enquire whether liberal-professional 'values' are 'real' or 'ersatz' is to miss the point. They have the capacity to be either or both, and in any particular situation they can and will be observed thus depending on the interpretations of the observers as well as the intent of the communicators. For child-care professionals, the scope is there for them to conceive of – and present – an act as protecting the child *or* as respecting the privacy of the family *or* as a symptom of stress or disillusion with the job, and the means by which choices are understood, made and defended is crucial to pursue. Even the governing concept of both British and French child-care law, the 'interest of the child', is riddled with ambiguity, itself representing a battleground for the advocates of rival interpretations. As in the case of Barthes's soldier, we may interpret the concept naïvely, cynically or mythically, as central to the issue of family regulation:

> 'The interest of the child', as a judicial criterion, is only apparently indefinable and empty. To the extent that it functions as a device for decision making this 'key concept' must be invested with at least sufficient weight that decisions do not appear purely gratuitous and arbitrary. That is what legitimates judicial intervention – the authority of the

judiciary itself as institution. It is not a question of denouncing 'the interest of the child' as a mask, an alibi, or a discourse tacked on to a legal process which in fact operates under different premises. Rather one must seek to discover the values and images which inform the criterion in a particular context and the specific processes of regulation implied by its use.

(Thèry 1989: 82)

In this chapter we have traversed the following points. First, we stated our premiss that secure accommodation is an aspect of child care and cannot be understood otherwise. Secondly, child care is an important corner of the relation between state and family. Thirdly, these relations have changed historically and in a sequence of mutations which has thrown the historians into confusion. Part of the source of this confusion is that the relations have changed because the phenomena they are linking have changed: so as the state is (self-evidently) not the same in twentieth-century Britain as it was in thirteenth-century France, nor is the family, nor the notion of childhood.

Fourthly, our brief consideration of the historians of childhood led us to identify a number of themes to be encountered again as we proceed. It is impossible to divorce the relations of state, family and child from the class structure of the society under consideration: the social role of the child is mediated by class membership, and this mediation profoundly affects the interaction of child and state.

Fifthly, the increasing interventions of the state in family life have been, perhaps as a piece of self-evident legitimation, through the offices of designated 'experts' – the pedagogues of the seventeenth century, the philanthropists and moralists of the eighteenth and nineteenth centuries and the clinical and 'welfare' experts of the twentieth century. It has not been our intention to evaluate the credentials of these experts but to understand the processes by which successions of them create and enforce their versions of 'normality', and how these endeavours impact on the lives and perceptions of the recipients of their expertise. Hence our interest in the conjunction of circumstances by which the family becomes increasingly private at the very time the state's salaried experts become more prolific, powerful and inquisitive.

Sixthly, we have introduced the framework of needs, rights and interests as constitutive of secure accommodation in this particular advanced liberal democracy. If we are correct in regarding secure accommodation neither naïvely nor cynically, the conventional analytic approach to it becomes a logical and conceptual impossibility: it is not our aim to *create* a synthesis so much as to *comprehend* the variety of possible syntheses with which the interplay of these concepts presents us.

Now this approach could itself be perceived as naïve, as though we were missing some clever strategy, conspiracy even, some subtle deceit of which the insiders are all too aware. Of course those engaged with secure accommodation are no less strategic, self-seeking or manipulative than those engaged in any other enterprise; but our aim is to address the self-evident reality that secure accommodation is different both from the penal establishments into which some children are placed *and* from the open establishments in which other children live.

Finally, underpinning our analysis is a theory, which we have described as cumulative, which led us to question the 'substitutive' analysis of Ariès (implying that one set of dominant beliefs replaces another), the implicit theory of stasis presented by Pollock (implying that *plus ça change, plus c'est la même chose*) and the idea of 'value perspectives' developed by Harding (implying that we can, against the evidence cited in the book itself, proceed on the assumption that people choose among and follow predetermined value positions). We confronted these views by using the notion of logocentrism, challenging the discourse which assumes there is a central explanatory principle. Logocentrism leads us to talk of objects rather than relations, to assume stasis when the world is spinning so very unpredictably. Once freed from the tyranny of the either–or, however, we can better engage with the paradoxes we encounter, paradoxes which are by no means always confusions to be eliminated by managerial decree or the application of rationality, but which sometimes actually move us closer to the totality of the experience. It is this theory of cumulation which provides part of the conceptual logic for the ambiguity of secure accommodation, which helps us comprehend this integration of needs, rights and interests and which explains the sub-title of this book in general and the 'thereabouts' in particular.

3 Young devils . . . or angels with dirty faces?

> In most societies in world history, the meaning of one's life has derived to a large degree from one's relationship to the lives of one's parents and one's children. For highly individuated Americans, there is something anomalous about the relation between parents and children, for the biologically normal dependence of children on adults is perceived as morally abnormal.
>
> (Bellah *et al.* 1985: 82)

> As a family we were too easily 'dared', as the phrase went, to attempt things dangerous or ridiculous. We were of Walter Bagehot's opinion that the greatest pleasure in life is doing what people say you cannot do, and the consequence was that we were often an anxiety to our parents, and often, owing to bodily damage, an affliction to ourselves.
>
> (John Buchan 1940: 31)

We turn now to the management of juvenile delinquents as it relates both to that of children we shall term 'needy' (youngsters classified as 'care or protection cases'), and to that of adult criminals. Clearly, all three of these fields, like the relationship between them, has changed considerably over time. Our approach turns mainly on the analytically key notion of 'juvenile delinquency'. How contemporary society deals with that form of juvenile behaviour which, to distinguish it from adult crime while maintaining some sense of culpability we term 'delinquency', can tell us much about contemporary views of childhood. It is because juvenile delinquents inhabit this no man's land between the pathetic and the wicked, between the voluntarism which neo-classical criminology conventionally affords most adult criminals and the helplessness, even innocence, which popular and professional perspectives afford the 'needy' child or the child-as-victim, that the manner in which the contemporary state deals with them is so instructive. If most delinquents can be perceived as naughty, as victims of circumstance or as both simultaneously, the manner in which they are processed tells us much about contemporary images of childhood and the family.

If juvenile delinquency occupies this bridging position between the loci of neediness and criminality, the question of how the *individual* juvenile delinquent is to be processed is key. Is it possible to conceive of an *operational* concept of delinquency which embraces both need and criminality, or is it necessary to proceed in more fragmented traditional fashion by sorting delinquents into needy sheep and criminal goats (see, for example, Rushforth 1978: ch. 6; Packman 1981: ch. 6)?

At this point we must reintroduce those 'experts', mainly social workers, one of whose functions it is to 'define reality', to justify by professional criteria the signification to be afforded a given delinquent. Our interest does not lie in the details of the professional discourse – how this debate is conducted by the experts – but in the nature and existence of the discourse itself, its social function, indeed necessity. Our point is akin to that of Foucault on madness, though devoid of Gallic passion:

> *We have yet to write the history of that other form of madness, by which men, in an act of sovereign reason, confine their neighbors, and communicate and recognize each other through the merciless language of non-madness . . . . None of the concepts of psychopathology, even and especially in the implicit process of retrospections, can play an organizing role. What is constitutive is the action that divides madness, and not the science elaborated once this division is made and calm restored.*
>
> (Italics original. Foucault 1971: xi)

To study how the immature are incarcerated, not exactly as criminals but on the basis of factors which relate to their actions as well as their youthful status, is especially illuminating. Secure accommodation is a particular form of 'locking up' which stands not primarily as 'custody' but, ironically, as an alternative to that more punitive intervention. When the title *Locking Up Children* (Millham *et al.* 1978) was chosen for the Dartington study as a stark reminder of what secure accommodation, stripped of euphemism, 'meant'[1] it was perhaps a necessary corrective to the sanitised discourse which designated secure accommodation a kind of self-protective moral hospital. This necessity, however, is no more. To the extent that it holds people where generally they do not wish to be, secure accommodation is, of course, coercive; but it is not *simply* coercive. True, it provides security for the rest of us *from* a child; yet it is also a form of security *for* a child, a safe boundary. It is here we differ from the Dartington researchers: to them secure accommodation is primarily punishment *disguised as* care; to us, however cynically it may on occasions be used, it 'is' both simultaneously, neither hospital nor prison but between the two – or thereabouts.

TOWARDS A LITERARY ANALYSIS: DRAMA AND NARRATIVE IN SOCIAL WORK

There are few certainties in the social world, and though there may be common-sense agreement as to the 'nature of truth' in a particular place at a particular time it is not strictly 'truth' which is agreed upon but a shared construction of 'meaning'.

This point emerged in Chapter 2 in relation to Pollock's study of adults' and children's diaries, and it represents a major problem in historiography. Our language and concepts are historically specific, and even what seem to us timeless categorisations of knowledge, belief or social formation are often less secure than that:

> We are so accustomed to classifying judgments, arguments and deeds in terms of morality that we forget how relatively new the notion was in the culture of the Enlightenment . . . . In Latin, as in ancient Greek, there is *no* word correctly translated by our word 'moral'. . . 'moralis', like its Greek predecessor '*êthikos*'. . . means 'pertaining to character' where a man's character is nothing other than his set dispositions to behave systematically in one way rather than another, to lead one particular kind of life.
>
> (MacIntyre 1981: 37)

Hence:

> Surely there have been individuals, and even whole societies, of whom and of which we would want to say that moral principles did not play any large part in their lives . . . . Homer, in approving the ferocity, guile and panache of the warrior chieftain, might well be said to have been employing moral standards different from our own; but he might just as well, or both, be said not to have been employing moral standards at all.
>
> (Warnock 1967: 54)

The 'family' too has, as we have also seen in Chapter 2, changed fundamentally over time. In medieval France, 'family' or *mesnie* stood in contradistinction to 'line', existing only for relatively brief periods and in noble families as an unstable form of joint ownership, ever vulnerable to a tightening of lineal solidarity. When the *mesnie* disintegrated (its main function of providing protection no longer being necessary), it subdivided into smaller units, with the line retaining its rights over the property given to members of the family. In the case of the peasantry, meanwhile, the 'family unit' was a less central organisational or economic unit than the community as a whole. Indeed the 'family' was generally less important to the phenomenology of people's worlds than now (Ariès 1962: 355), yet the form of the discourse reported by historians such as Pollock appears to have shifted less than the content. The denotation 'family' is constant, but its connotation has changed beyond recognition.

If we are 'in and of the moment that we are attempting to analyse, in and of the structures we employ to analyse it' (Connor 1989: 5), it is not merely involvement which gets in the way of 'objectivity'. The meaning structures by which we 'make sense of' cultural experiences are themselves part of that culture. Even the notions that there *is* a culture, that we *can* 'step outside' it, that there *is* an 'I' existing outside of culture but vulnerable to penetration by self-will or some kind of essentialist psychology, are strictly culture-bound. For how, ultimately, can we 'know' that such notions exist when our means of 'knowing' are themselves the products of culture?[2]

Thus far we have examined the changing 'natures' of family and childhood as they reflect these awkward conjunctions of private family and interventive state; children as increasingly 'liberated' from property status yet unable to exercise all the 'rights' which others claim for them; children as oppressed or confused or in some other way helpless, yet simultaneously powerful, having potential for evil, needing to be tamed. Secure accommodation represents one of the state's ultimate responses to this problem nexus. It is not simply a matter of punishing conscious and calculated crimes committed by juveniles, for secure accommodation is a disposal precisely 'without' a centre, situated somewhere 'between' hospital and prison, and containing youngsters 'between' sickness and wickedness, for whose circumstance no word exists in the English language, no concept 'behind' the language and no alternative administrative facility.

To have 'no centre' is, however, perceptually difficult in contemporary western culture, and is liable to herald a struggle for hegemony among competing groups. In our sphere of interest the struggles have been intermittently passionate disputes about the sovereignty of needs, rights or interests, the nature of 'care', the means by which the state can (or should) provide 'security' for the troubled or family-less child, and what constitutes the proper action of the state when faced with sometimes extreme forms of youthful deviance. All these considerations turn, however, on the notion that in one corner there is 'need' and in the other 'crime', separate commodities requiring, in Harding's word, 'balancing'.

Child-care experts, themselves part of the culture from which this dualism emerges, are charged with attempting a reconciliation of these differences, with selecting from the range of legally acceptable actions the one which appears most 'suitable' in a particular case. Whilst the knowledge on which such judgements are based is not 'scientific' in the Popperian sense of being open to refutation, nor is it necessarily 'false'. Doubtless we can say with hindsight that a certain decision or action was wise or not, proper or not, successful or not, but we can seldom say that *therefore* we will do the same thing again because we shall never again meet exactly the 'same' situation in which to do it.

Human service professions such as social work, in contradistinction to more technical professions, constitute rather uncertain habitations for formal 'theory' or 'knowledge' (Sibeon 1991). There actions derive from a cluster of professional considerations such as experience, professional values, agency socialisation, individual interest, commitment and hunch, and such subterranean ambitions as the quest for an easy life and the desire to impress one's superiors. The transfer of experience, though indispensable if sense is to be made of the work, is inevitably a little 'hit and miss'. This makes prediction difficult if not impossible:

> For the central function of the social scientist as expert advisor or manager is to predict the outcomes of alternative policies, and if his predictions do not derive from a knowledge of law-like generalisations, the status of the social scientist as predictor becomes endangered – as, so it turns out, it ought to be; for the record of social scientists as predictors is very bad indeed.
>
> (MacIntyre 1981: 85)

This theoretical vacuum existing in the 'social' professions (Donzelot 1984; Harris and Webb 1987: 66–9) has been largely filled by a mode of explanation we term 'narrative'. A thread of literary interest exists in the social work discourse in particular. This has in the past been expressed as a simple belief that to read fine literature will heighten social workers' sensitivity to their clientele and provide new insights into the human condition (see, for example, Morris 1975; Irvine 1982; Valk 1983). Indeed, social work has itself been seen as an 'art' (England 1986) and literature a mode of social enquiry into intimate areas where respondent resistance may sabotage more conventional research methods (Wilson and Ridler 1989).

Our interest is different, though related. We too believe in a connection between literature and life, but in a stronger, more integral sense. First, we take account of aspects of post-structuralist and postmodernist cultural and literary theory; secondly, we are interested in the notion of social work as a dramatic intervention, and introduce it in this chapter. Thirdly, and more extensively, we are concerned to explore how narrative can help explicate the work of the professionals (for an earlier consideration of which see also Whan 1979). One of us has elsewhere used Alasdair MacIntyre's idea of the 'narrative self' (MacIntyre 1981: ch. 15) to illuminate aspects of adoption practice (Haimes and Timms 1985), but MacIntyre's work has value beyond any specialist area. Of conversation, for example, he observes:

> The use of words such as 'tragic', 'comic', and 'farcical' is not marginal to such evaluations. We allocate conversations to genres, just as we do literary narratives. Indeed a conversation is a literary work, even if a very short one, in which the participants are not only the actors, but also the joint authors, working out in agreement or disagreement the mode of their production . . . . But if this is true of conversations, it is true also *mutatis mutandis* of battles, chess games, courtships, philosophy seminars, families at the dinner table, businessmen negotiating contracts – that is, of human interactions in general. For conversation, understood widely enough, is the form of human transactions in general.
>
> (MacIntyre 1981: 196–7)

Art by no means acts as a mere 'mirror' on life (as naturalist authors and critics would have it), but art, the medium in which it is expressed and our understanding of 'life' itself all derive from the same culture and history, all coexist in interrelated manner, all are rendered intelligible by the same cultural, aesthetic, intellectual and moral processes. Neither 'life' nor 'art' as we understand them can quite exist without the other, and as art is 'part of' life, so is life 'part of' art. Goffman and the symbolic interactionists have so precisely followed Shakespeare in demonstrating that all the world's a stage (and the men and women merely actors) that they make this latter point for us perfectly. Raymond Williams, in his aptly named *Drama in a Dramatised World*, offers further clarification:

> Our present society, in ways it is merely painful to reiterate, is sufficiently dramatic in one obvious sense. Actions of a kind and scale that attract dramatic comparisons are being played out in ways that leave us continually uncertain whether we are spectators or participants. The specific vocabulary of the dramatic mode – drama itself, and then tragedy, scenario, situation, actors, performances, roles, images – is continually and conventionally appropriated for these immense actions.
>
> (Williams 1975: 13)

Social experts characteristically operate in self-consciously dramatic spheres – courts and prisons, the enclosed private spaces inhabited by people at the centre of some dramatic episode of crime or tragedy. It is this which makes drama such a powerful motif for the social worker's professional world. Part of the drama doubtless stems from anthropological curiosity, even prurience, among the social workers themselves, few of whom seem to lack either inquisitiveness or an enthusiasm for engaging in that paradoxical activity best termed confidential gossiping, which derives professional sanction from the idea that it is a necessary means of gaining 'support' in stressful situations. More significantly, however, the curtain rising on the scene of professional intervention is the very stuff of drama. The social worker enters the enclosed space of the client's front room, the client enters the social-work office, the social worker rings the secure unit doorbell and the manager opens it, offers tea and biscuits and begins to talk. In each of these situations the character is metaphorically walking on to the set, and we know a drama is about to unfold.

Certain features of social work, therefore, make it especially 'dramatic'. It is primarily a verbal, but sometimes a physical, interaction taking place in territory which is frequently the setting for drama[3], and it occurs at moments which are themselves dramatic. Dramatic conventions exist too, as they do in all 'conversations', but in characteristically heightened form: there is dramatic 'space' between the actors, expressed in terms of differential 'knowledge', class and power; dramatic 'distance', expressed as different levels of involvement; and dramatic 'irony' as the 'wise' professional sees all too well but is often unable to circumvent the trap which the 'unwise' client is setting for himself. We shall see examples of these phenomena in Chapter 5.

Part of social work's dramatic character is that because it is 'real' it does not necessarily follow the formulaic pathways of popular fiction or drama wherein all tensions are resolved, for better or worse, by the final page or curtain. The affirmations of justice, dignity and resilience daily celebrated in popular fiction and mass theatre need not 'come true' in the world of social work: injustices may continue, needs may not be met, interests may be ignored and rights abrogated. Even more characteristically, nothing may be resolved. The comforting predictability of the popular arts, characteristically signalled even before we buy the book or enter the theatre by 'signs' ranging from the design of dust wrappers to the tone and content of publicity blurbs, is altogether missing in the social worker's world.

Narrative does have uses for the social professionals, for the day-to-day experience of playing protagonist in dramas which often go wrong has its psychological consequences. The cognitive dissonance resulting from experiencing yet being all too often unable to close the gap between the dramatic imperative of predictable outcome and the experience of not necessarily failure but incompleteness can be reduced by the use of narrative. When we tell stories we mould and remould messy 'reality' into a comprehensible shape: people take on familiar roles, encounter familiar obstacles, triumph or fail for reasons which become reassuringly clear. Such reasons confirm individual and cultural stereotypes, reinforcing our pre-existing world view, albeit in necessarily modified form, making sense of the otherwise inexplicable. So, through the creative and reconstitutive process of narrative, failure may come to be experienced as resulting from the conduct of a created but recognisable 'villain' – an unsympathetic social security official, a pompous clerk of the court, a remote director of social services, a recalcitrant 'client' – or merely be the result of an unjust world or sheer bad luck. Memory creates as well as recalls, and, whether or not the analysis is 'true' it offers a means of structuring and comprehending 'reality' and, because it determines the manner of necessary interpretation, becomes part of that 'reality'. Such a cognitive and creative process is, of course, not restricted to social workers:

> 'Fact' is in modern culture a folk-concept with an aristocratic ancestry. When Lord Chancellor Bacon. . . enjoined his followers to abjure speculation and collect facts, he was immediately understood by such as John Aubrey to have identified facts as collectors' items . . . Aubrey's error was of course not only to suppose that the natural scientist is a kind of magpie; it was also to suppose that the observer can confront a fact face-to-face without any theoretical interpretation interposing itself.
>
> (MacIntyre 1981: 76)

If natural scientists, albeit sometimes unbeknown to themselves, cannot but tell stories it is unsurprising that social workers do so too. Indeed, the language of the theatre spills into their professional jargon: their training includes 'role play'; their clients are said to 'act out' their problems; in their day-to-day discussions they speak of people in 'crisis'; they advise people on how to 'dress up' for court, 'prompting' them on what to say and how to behave. They 'rehearse' them for job interviews; they record and, like a Greek chorus, comment on the day-to-day human tragedy and comedy of the lives of marginal, vulnerable, impulsive and unpredictable people. And, through their job, the social workers receive temporary, honorary membership of this nether world, one in which they may become emotionally, intellectually and personally, but never totally or permanently, involved.

In short, we see the experts, with a professional preference for oral tradition and narrative over theory and analysis, occupying the territory of drama, struggling to make sense of a painful, exciting, fundamentally ambiguous and unpredictable world, but one in which they have frequently to take decisive and significant action.

We must, however, beware of implying false homogeneity in our use of literary and narrative devices: there is, after all, literature and literature – classics and trash (Hawkins 1990). Classic literature, both traditional and avant-garde, has about it a 'terrorist' potential with which the 'critically conscious' reader must engage (Docherty 1987). More recent forms of terrorist literature characteristically lack the certainty provided by the guiding hand of a writer whose 'author-ity' steers readers in a predetermined direction, challenging them instead to engage in an active mode of reading which, because it is fundamentally creative, is largely indistinguishable from the process of authorship. Hence Umberto Eco's section head 'How to produce texts by reading them' (Eco 1979: 3) and the contemporary critical view that the text is the product of its own reciprocal relation with the reader. Having as it does unwritten as well as written dimensions, the text's omissions are potentially as significant as its inclusions, and lacking as it does any objectively definable and agreed facticity, text and reader coexist in an internal economy of their own creation, an economy which possesses its own intellectual and aesthetic imperatives:

> Just as the reader participates in the production of the text's meaning so the text shapes the reader. On the one hand it 'selects' its appropriate reader, projects an image of such a reader, through its specific linguistic code, its style . . . . On the other hand, just as the text pre-shapes a certain competence to be brought by the reader from the outside, so in the course of reading, it developes [*sic*] in the reader a specific competence needed to come to grips with it, often inducing him to change his previous conceptions and modify his outlook. The reader is thus both an image of a certain competence brought to the text and a structuring of such a competence within the text.
>
> (Rimmon-Kenan 1983: 117–18)

Trash, on the other hand, is formulaic literature, dubbed 'an alternative "holiday-hospital" for women' (Fowler 1991: 171; see Eco 1979: ch. 4 for a similar consideration of Superman as sating a 'hunger for redundance'), and can be studied more systematically than classics because it is both predictable and safe.[4] The same, perhaps, applies to other modes of formulaic literature which, for historical and cultural reasons, must be treated less pejoratively. For example, Vladimir Propp's seminal study of the structure and motifs of folk tales (Propp 1928) analysed the action as containing thirty-one 'functions', or significant actions. In Propp's formulation, any one folk tale would contain a range of these functions in much the same sequence,[5] invariably ending with the exposure and punishment of the villain (or false hero) and the marriage and accession of the true hero.

This literary tension between on the one hand the formulaic and predictable and on the other the terrorist has a particular application in the world of the professionals. It is a common experience for neophyte professionals in particular to be amazed at how different 'the same' events seem when recounted by different participants, different narrators – the warring husband and wife, the offender and the policeman, the defence and the prosecution. Yet typically neither party is lying, but offering different perspectives, engaging in different modes of presentation, following different scripts, playing different parts.[6] We all, when we hear a tale of individual heroics, whether it is of the little man making good or of the devotion of a household pet, have a seemingly 'natural' response based on culturally shared conventions. It is as the tale becomes more complex and detailed that these responses become more divergent, when we deal, for example, with the duplicity of the deserving and the sadness of the undeserving. Increasing complexity shifts us from the realms of 'trash' to the more ambiguous world of classics. Great art presents us with moral dilemmas, problems of action, ontological doubts of just the kind we have in mind in discussing the problems which face the professionals.

It is the idea that it falls to the professionals to treat as complex and ambiguous situations which others may see stereotypically that drives our considerations in this chapter. We must not, however, take our analogy too far. When Gaston Dominici, a poor farmer aged 80, was condemned in 1952 for the murder of Sir Jack Drummond and his family, the words used at the trial were, appropriately given our analysis, those of high drama:

> it is in the name of a 'universal' psychology that old Dominici has been condemned: descending from the charming empyrean of bourgeois novels and essentialist psychology, Literature has just condemned a man to the guillotine. Listen to the Public Prosecutor: '*Sir Jack Drummond, I told you, was afraid. But he knows that in the end the best way to defend oneself is to attack. So he throws himself on this fierce-looking man and takes the old man by the throat. Not a word is spoken. But to Gaston Dominici, the simple fact that someone should want to hold him down by both shoulders is unthinkable. It was physically impossible for him to bear this strength which was suddenly pitted against him.*' This is credible like the temple of Sesostris, like the Literature of M. Genevoix. Only, to base archaeology or the novel on a 'Why not?' does not harm anybody. But Justice?
>
> (Barthes 1973: 48–9)

A TALE OF TWO TALES: THE DEVILS AND THE ANGELS

> Swamji turned back toward me, cheeks lifted under their white stubble in a toothless and delighted grin . . . . 'Educated people always doubt everything. They lie awake at night thinking, "What was that? Why did it happen? What is the meaning and the cause of it?" Uneducated people pass judgment and walk on. They get a good night's sleep.'
>
> (Narayan 1989: 2–3)

> Can you imagine John Wayne playing a character with a first-hand knowledge of the works of Christopher Marlowe?
>
> (Hawkins 1990: 13)

So there is literature and literature. Only a limited number of fictional types are available to story-tellers, albeit endlessly recycled within certain traditions, every 'plot' comprising a unique set of variations on a theme (Tambling 1991). Popular literature, both oral and written, has characteristically sought to be predictable rather than surprising (except, of course, within bounds which are themselves strictly conventional), consoling rather than disturbing. Hence Brecht's reference to popular culture as 'a branch of the capitalist narcotics industry' and Horkheimer's claim that the masses reject the avant-garde because it is disturbing to their unthinking acquiescence in their own oppression (cited in Selden 1985: 34); or, in the homelier perspective of the early Arnold Bennett, 'A fine book is above the populace; if the populace reaches up to it let us praise the populace' (Bennett 1901: 172). To Gramsci (in his *Prison Notebooks*) popular literature must offer a collective representation of the sentiments of the 'silent multitude': hence were Dumas's readers 'intoxicated' by his characters' capacity to demonstrate the continued existence of a justice which they suspected no longer existed (cited in Fowler 1991: 31). Similarly, both nineteenth-century detective novels and twentieth-century science fiction offer the consoling thought that order and logic can be restored to a world troubled by the devastation of war, the (seemingly) constant threat of revolution and the intellectually sobering realisation, based on relativity and quantum physics, that the very structure of the universe is mutable, unpredictable, random and, since Heisenberg's Uncertainty Principle, unmeasurable.

Part of the social, political and psychological function of great art is anarchic: to disturb, break rules, offend, question, while popular art contents itself with placating, playing with the emotions, pretending to fulfil dreams. Popular literature provides security through predictability and order; it reinforces conventional expectations of family and gender but also requires the characters to have emotional, class and political contact with the readers. So a sample of working-class female Scottish readers repudiated Barbara Cartland on political, and Jackie Collins on moral and psychological, grounds (Collins's pulp novel *Hollywood Wives* apparently transgressing 'too deeply their moral categories, destroying their careful resistance to passions perceived as animal-like or exploitative' [Fowler 1991: 174]). Catherine Cookson, on the other hand, in combining the traditions of conventional romance and working-class fiction, was overwhelmingly popular: 'Thus there is evidence that lower-class readers *do select* those writers whose portrayals of the world both pinpoint some elements of their own alienation and whose hopes express their own aspirations' (Fowler 1991: 174).

The century which has witnessed such an increase in working-class literature has also, of course, witnessed a development of 'intellectual' art through modernists (Joyce, Woolf, Eliot, Yeats) and postmodernists (Eco, Beckett, Barth, Olson, Fowles) (for an explanation of these distinctions see, for example, Connor 1989). This has, if nothing else, sustained the social role of the book as a ticket to class membership. Whereas, however, the conflict between the popular and intellectual novel was stark in the modernist era (see, for example, Virginia Woolf's notorious attack on Arnold Bennett in *Mr Bennett and Mrs Brown*) (Woolf 1924), more recently there has been concern to bridge the two. Leslie Fiedler in particular, in an influential essay 'Cross that border – close that gap' (Fiedler 1971) argued precisely that the generic integrity of 'high culture' should be challenged. Many contemporary postmodernist texts are written in more accessible language while still engaging in the self-conscious introspection, intertextuality – or, in the phrase of one critic, narcissism (Hutcheon 1984) – and ontological enquiry so characteristic of the genre. *Foucault's Pendulum* (Eco 1989) suffices as an example of what Linda Hutcheon terms intertextual metafiction: a book about a book, containing themes ranging from the quest for the Grail, the structure of the universe and the nature of being, love and betrayal to the nature, purpose and potential of the new technology; and using as method a combination of picaresque plot construction, schoolboy humour and tightly structured and arcane scholarship. And in yet another postmodernist paradox the post-structuralist critic David Lodge publishes humorous novels which, while they play a number of intellectual games with their readers, are essentially formulaic.[7]

Similarly, in the world of art and film the work of Andy Warhol is the apotheosis of intellectually aspirant populism, involving the creation of 'art' out of (literally) trash, but art which has nothing 'behind' it. With Warhol no decoding is possible, for his work expresses precisely the indissolubility of art and trash in a world which worships the tinsel image, the motor bike or the convenience food. In the world of television, the logic of *Twin Peaks* derives from its very intertextuality, almost every scene being a pastiche of something else. How do we categorise such a mode? Not, surely, as merely offering scope for literary detective work at dinner parties, its allusions superfluous to its creative purpose; but nor, certainly, as great art, deriving its poetics from its metafictional structure, its allusions fundamental aspects of its purpose – rather as we might say of T.S. Eliot's *The Waste Land*.

Twin Peaks bridges the gap between high and low art. In its self-consciously parodic style it is laughing both at itself and, inextricably, at the mode of which it is a part. While it can, therefore, be 'read' as 'straight' *or* as 'parody', in its central aesthetic it is both simultaneously.[8] Rather as the alternative endings of John Fowles's postmodernist novel *The French*

Lieutenant's Woman (Fowles 1969) do not make it *either* happy *or* sad precisely because the fact that the reader can 'choose' transforms both happiness and sadness into something different from each, so in *Twin Peaks* does the coexistence of straightness and parody lead to the transformation of both into something which is neither.[9]

As we have argued, the 'real' world too has about it a complexity and unpredictability, even anarchy, which does not lend itself to formulaic modes. Yet it is in such modes that we perceive fragments of 'reality' as they are daily served up in the verbal conversations of family, friends, acquaintances and broadcasters and in the written conversations of the press. Whilst the blurring of classic and formulaic modes in much post-modern art may lead us to question any simple division of literature into popular and complex (see in particular Hawkins 1990 for a discussion of the mutual indebtedness of popular writers and classicists), our purpose is to show how 'simple' motifs are transformed into more complex ones. The truism that the more we know the more we know we do not know illumines the awkward function of the social expert of not merely simplifying and solving problems but of complicating that which was once straightforward. This is the function of the artist too.

We tell in this book, therefore, a tale of two tales, observing what happens when they collide, when a choice must be made between two incompatible forms, the heroic and the moral, the potential victim struggling to defeat the machine which threatens to crush him and the miscreant whose misdeeds create misery among the innocent being rightly punished. For it is precisely with this clash of two irreconcilable scripts that the social professionals are called on to deal. As we have seen, however, the raw material with which they engage, being characteristically complex and ambiguous, has few of the qualities of formulaic fiction. Part of the experts' job is to comprehend and express this complexity, creating precisely this synthesis which is a characteristic of classic literature.

Unfortunately, however, the interested parties with whom the social workers engage by no means necessarily wish to engage with this complexity. Typically courts, administrators, lawyers, press and public wish complexity to be 'filtered' so that the emerging narrative will make sense to *them*, will guide their actions with a decisiveness which belies and denies the existential dilemmas which together constitute the 'problem which has no answer'. Social professionals engage with, comprehend and process the raw materials of classic literature, yet transform them for public (or at least administrative) consumption into something simple and formulaic from which unambiguous action imperatives follow. How they make their choices, how pressures are brought to bear on them to transform phenomena which have no neat 'ending' into a piece of popular art – to have the work of Camus, perhaps, overwritten by Mr Mickey Spillane – is part of our theme too.

The numbers of available plots is, as we have seen, limited. Here we tell two of them. They are not the only two motifs available to us, but have been selected to express the awkward relation between criminality and deprivation with which those involved with secure accommodation are sanctioned to engage, and which they perpetually struggle to transcend. We tell our tales in simplified but we hope recognisable form: the first is a crime story of the young devils brought to justice, the second a moral tale of social injustice – the story of the angels with dirty faces. Both are formulaic, and it is central to our thesis that most youngsters in secure accommodation occupy a *locus* between these tales (or thereabouts), but in such a manner that they may, according to a range of extraneous and possibly even arbitrary factors, be assigned without difficulty to either.

Tale A: the young devils

The motif of this genre is instantly recognisable as formulaic fiction. Whether the story is of cops and robbers, cowboys and Indians, the *samurai* and the brigands or, for that matter, the expulsion of the rebel angels from Heaven, the elemental struggle between good and evil is a feature of popular literature in most, if not all, cultures.

Often the motif has a strong element of *cleansing*. The cleansing theme exists in a tradition stretching back through popular romance, some of which has subsequently been translated in sanitised form into children's literature (Robin Hood, William Tell, the Arthurian legends) through medieval Celtic tales (the *Mabinogion*), the Old English epics (*Beowulf*) and Icelandic sagas (*Njal's Saga*) to the ancient Greeks, the Old Testament and pagan mythology. As cultures have developed and societies become more complex, the nature of the cleansing has changed. We no longer have an omnipotent, avenging anthropomorphic deity wreaking havoc on Sodom and Gomorrah, nor yet, except in the modernist form of *The Waste Land*, the Fisher King regenerating the waste land with fertility. Though popular art contains its versions of these struggles, the moral categories are less clear, the heroes less pure, the villains more sympathetic. There is in much contemporary popular art a moral, cultural and hence artistic relativism which leads to the portrayal of these struggles in the self-consciously parodic form of, for example, James Bond or Batman.

The tradition has not, of course, been lost as much as modified into a literary framework congruent with contemporary forms of popular culture. The devils tradition proceeds, therefore, but in one of two main forms, and in this distinction lies a complexity to which we shall later return, for it has considerable impact on the professionals whose judgements and opinions we shall be discussing. The first form of the devils tradition is the Old Testament variety wherein the devil, be it Dr Faustus himself or one of his many close relations from Don Giovanni to Svengali, once apprehended suffers a form of permanent *exclusion* – if not by being dragged, literally, to Hell then by denunciation followed by death, mutilation, banishment or imprisonment. It is as though a retributive urge reflects some collective sense that the 'devil' concerned is to be defined as having gone beyond the pale, being irredeemable, having committed (literally or in secular metaphor) the unforgivable sin. The exclusion of the devils stems from a collective fear of contamination, a sense that if an example be not made of the miscreant the divide between good and evil will be riven, with the consequent destruction of the moral, social and political order – the stuff, in short, of Aristotelian tragedy.

There is also, however, a second, New Testament, form of the tale, culminating not in exclusion but in inclusion. In this form of the tradition the devil, seeing the error of his ways, repents, receives forgiveness and dedicates his life to the welfare of others. There are, though, constraints on this impulse to inclusivity, and the structures within which it occurs are not always free of equivocation or ambiguity, nor yet of the protective comfort of the exclusionary motif. So the religious order represents a half-way house between liberty and incarceration: 'Get thee to a nunnery!' has reformist as well as penitent and redemptive dimensions, yet also implies distance, remoteness and the security of the rules of the Order, the safety of the institution itself. The 'inclusionary' motif in literature is not, therefore, a withdrawal, but a displacement of power, a statement only partially or incidentally humane (Foucault 1977: 23) but reflecting the collective confidence of a society in its capacity to control and change that 'devil' who accordingly becomes something 'other than' a devil, a tame deviant, a symbol of the capacity of a mature society to contain rather than expel its own evil.

Tale B: the angels with dirty faces

The motif is borrowed, of course, from an inter-war Warner Brothers gangster film in which a gang of deprived youngsters becomes embroiled with racketeers before its members see the error of their ways. The genre has, however, a longer pedigree than that, for the tale is of juvenile distress, of waifs and water babies, of temporary estrangement from righteousness for what we would now call 'environmental reasons'. The theme is contamination, the poisoning of good by evil, and the genre involves reclaiming the good, relieving them of their misery and oppression. The reader, though, is no avenging angel, no Sir Gawain cleansing the land of green giants, but Mr Brownlow in search of an Oliver Twist.

This genre differs entirely from that of the young devils. When we read in a novel of a fictional child in distress, or in a newspaper of a real one – a child beaten, burned, missing or abducted – we immediately know which genre is involved and accordingly how to respond to the story. Just as in the world of fiction we cannot imagine Bram Stoker making a contribution to the works of Charles Kingsley, or Marie Corelli to those of Simone de Beauvoir, so we learn to distinguish the tale in the popular press of evil or horror from that of misery and goodness. If the headline tells us that a thief has stolen a charity box just before Christmas, thereby depriving handicapped children of the gifts on which the contents of the box were to be spent, certain emotions and beliefs are immediately evoked in us. And only the more intellectual readers – perhaps those not accustomed to reading the pulp novels of which this kind of story is the 'real life' counterpart – will wish to check those emotions, identify what is not said as well as what is, and consider whether the story could have been told differently – to engage, in short, in the act of generative, constitutive reading which we have been discussing.

If, however, we learn – either at the time or, more probably, later – that the thief in question has had a sad life, that there is in that life not, of course, a justification but an explanation, which entitles, even obliges, us to view him with compassion rather than contempt, we are engaging in a more complex form of moral evaluation than normally characterises popular art. Indeed, if we are unaccustomed to such dilemmas we may even round on those experts who complicate things thus, accusing them of offering feeble excuses or sociological alibis, even of condoning the act itself. Similarly, when faced with an exploited innocent we can play the part of Brownlow without difficulty, but when there is a hint of voluntarism – in the child prostitute, for example, who, spurning all attempts at reclamation, becomes incorrigible – we have a more complex problem.

Popular literature is, then, predictable and reassuring, and our interest in reading it is only superficially to learn the outcome (to discover, say, the identity of the murderer or the fate of the heroine). More fundamentally it is to enjoy the spectacle and the moral tale it tells. Hence to Eco, an Ian Fleming novel is precisely analagous to

> a game of basketball played by the Harlem Globetrotters against a local team. We know with absolute confidence that the Globetrotters will win; the pleasure lies in the trained virtuosity with which they defer the final moment, with what ingenious deviations they reconfirm the foregone conclusion, with what trickeries they make rings round their opponents. (Eco 1979: 160–1)

And popular fiction generally is akin to Barthes's account of professional wrestling as a spectacle whose outcome is never in doubt masquerading as a sport whose outcome is unknowable:

> Each sign in wrestling is therefore endowed with an absolute clarity, since one must always understand everything on the spot. As soon as the adversaries are in the ring, the public is overwhelmed with the obviousness of the roles. As in the theatre, each physical type expresses to excess the part which has been assigned to the contestant.
>
> (Barthes 1973: 17)

Popular literature sustains a range of culturally shared, or at least comprehensible, forms of explanation, present to varying degrees in the consciousness of most or all members of a culture, which contribute to a climate in which studied equivocation is avoided if not despised. The essence of all this human drama is that it is routine, and the representation of what is other-than-routine, which raises uncertainties which are most comfortably avoided, is disturbing. When we charge a group of experts with matters about which their understanding is sophisticated and detailed and ours superficial, when their version of the story is by Camus, ours by Spillane, we may become disturbed, incredulous, angry when our respective conclusions differ, when the simple answer we seek becomes instead a new dilemma necessitating moral or intellectual engagement with a difficulty which had never previously crossed our minds.

How, though, does this theorising relate to secure accommodation, child care and the management of delinquency? Are not these matters which occur in the 'real' world, not the realms of fiction? Is it not a luxury to write of fiction and not reality? We think not, for there *is* no clear divide between the understanding of the 'real' and the 'fictional'. Though our reference to the condemnation of Gaston Dominici signals an 'obvious' difference between the two, social actions and fiction derive from the same cultural norms, the same social philosophies. Each is generative not reflective, and the old saw about truth being stranger than fiction is a common-sense expression of this point. The 'actions' available in the world of fiction or drama ought to be infinite, transcending the universe, defying the laws of physics and biology, exceeding by far those available in reality to mere mortals. Yet they still end up as a small number of plots with only the names of the characters, the settings, the language changed. The rebel writer breaks these rules but within a short time becomes – as the modernists of the early twentieth century did – the establishment against which the next generation of rebels must pit itself. As Arnold Bennett, rejecting the romanticism of Victorian fiction, embraced the naturalism of Zola only to be repudiated by the modernist Virginia Woolf, so in turn did Woolf come to be attacked by some (though not all – see Moi 1985: 2–18) contemporary feminists for the primitive nature of her own feminism (for example, Showalter 1977; Lovell 1983), for her contradictions, her elitism, her snobbery. And, pathetically but interminably craving the esteem of others as she did, she knew her 'sink in the scale' (Woolf 1953: 231) would happen: the answer was, even then, to adopt a posture which made her look better than others:

> It is perhaps true that my reputation will now decline. I shall be laughed at and pointed at. What should be my attitude – clearly Arnold Bennett and Wells took the criticism of their youngers in the wrong way. The right way is not to resent; not to be longsuffering and Christian and submissive either. Of course, with my odd mixture of extreme rashness and modesty [*sic*] (to analyse roughly) I very soon recover from praise and blame. But I want to find out an attitude. The most important thing is not to think very much about oneself [*sic*].
>
> (Woolf 1953: 180)

Social actors, then, like creative writers, operate within rules and traditions (Eliot 1919; MacIntyre 1981), and though to shift paradigms is first to be 'creative' and 'innovative', it is then to set new rules which come to be incorporated in an existing tradition. The factors which make literature fashionable, acceptable, trash or classic are those that determine which social actions are 'acceptable', 'progressive', 'fair'. When social workers look at a 'case', what they see is not 'the case' in all its objective starkness, but a particular representation which draws on what Foucault calls the cultural archive, the positive Unconscious (Selden 1985: 101), as well as on those more personal tactics of classification used at varying levels of consciousness to make sense of new situations. So in a new situation we fall back on our personal reservoir of experience and ask: What does the incident, the situation, the person even, remind me of? Is the individual to be trusted? What is my construction of these various disconnected pieces of 'knowledge'? Each 'case' is a story waiting to be told, and the fact that the pain and pleasure which appear in that story are 'real' does not make it less of a story.

One of the means by which the true stories of complex humanity are transmitted into popular fiction is that self-imposed and self-justifying arbiter of popular morality, the tabloid press[10] (see also Soothill and Walby 1991). Tales of villains sell newspapers, partly, no doubt, for prurient reasons but partly too because the popular press is so accomplished at turning messy reality into simple, recognisable, moral tales. 'LET HIM STARVE!' screamed a headline in one tabloid paper following the imprisonment of a man who starved his daughter to death, over a piece which, by blending a court report with an animadversion on liberal penal policy, constituted a perfect editorialisation of the news story. And where policy proposals of this kind seem inappropriate, the tendency is to demand a collective attitudinal change among members of those occupational groups charged with setting an example to others – teachers, psychiatrists, social workers, Anglican bishops – though seldom, surprisingly enough, the owners or employees of the tabloid press itself.

Popular fiction characteristically objectifies its subjects. We seldom encounter a Raskolnikov or a Lord Jim in the popular press or pulp novel, and though as we have seen even in formulaic fiction the clear boundaries of right and wrong have become attenuated, it remains rare for the villain to be wracked with guilt or sorrow, or the hero with *Angst.* It is central to the genre that the devils are clearly mad or bad, lacking in reason or relentless in the pursuit of evil. On the rare occasions that we are permitted to hear the villain's tale – be the villain moors murderer, football hooligan or IRA terrorist – we are usually informed editorially that the tale itself confirms either madness or badness. The more poorly put together the tale, the more likely the devil is to be portrayed as mad, the more lucid and cogent, the more plausibly he can be presented as the very embodiment of evil.[11]

So it is that those whose task it is to interpret the devil's story create an unease in others which may have repercussions for how they do their job. It is the classics, not trash, which say the unsayable, which break the rules, which show the interrelationship of good and bad: but to expose these complexities to a public bred on pulp is not without its frustrations and indeed dangers.

ENTER THE EXPERTS: EXPLAINERS AND EXCUSERS

Part of the function of experts is to make sense of the otherwise unintelligible (Harris and Webb 1987), albeit on the basis of imperfect judgement and fallible knowledge, and often on the brink of a chasm of uncertainty. The point is by no means that the 'experts' in this sphere have privileged access to the fundamental truths of human behaviour or that they possess some arcane technical capacity (akin to that of the civil engineer, microbiologist or nuclear physicist). On the contrary, they regularly encounter situations beyond the scope of their influence; their expertise frequently fails to find a pathway through the thicket. The forms of knowledge available to the social experts often complicate rather than simplify matters, and the consequences of this complexification can all too easily surface as professional hesitancy if not immobility. This in turn is usually incomprehensible to the laity who not only, at least in western cultures, look to experts to produce answers, but who may well see the issue as rather simple.

Social professionals act in situations which are ambiguous precisely because it is in such situations that they are needed: one does not need an expert to do simple things. When the professionals meet an Oliver who, though he has no Brownlow to save him, has no Sykes to corrupt him either – a sad and disadvantaged boy, true, but one who also shows every intention of, as it were, continuing to steal the pocket handkerchieves – difficult choices have to be made. The situation is complex, the moral choice hard. Law and policy can seldom give firm guidance, and it is not often that there is an administrative solution which reflects the complexity of the problem: for all the refinement of the analysis, what can be done is restricted to what is available. The ultimate choice can, therefore, indeed be between the scripts of our two 'simple' tales, turning on the question of whether some new Oliver Twist is a young devil or an angel with a dirty face, and failing to address the greater complexities involved. Yet even this choice is not easy: doubtless much of the remarkable defensiveness of many social professionals about the tabloid press is based on the fear of choosing one story and being pilloried for not choosing the other.

Professionals reading this will perhaps protest: of course they must transcend stereotypes and live with complexity; and anyway decisions on these matters are not theirs but belong to the judges and magistrates whom they simply advise. This latter point is formally correct but partial; because it is important, however, we deal with it here analytically, and approach it empirically in Chapter 6, when we show the practical impact of the advice of the experts on decision making. One cannot after all be simultaneously a humble adviser and an expert to be taken note of without some room for confusion creeping in.

The idea that the experts act as 'advisers' to the court in, for example, difficult child-care cases falsely implies that they maintain a studied detachment from the drama. In reality, however, the experts are important actors, strategists with their own views as to what should happen, persuaders as well as advisers. We know, from a substantial literature on the reports they write for courts, for example (reviewed in Harris 1992: ch. 7), that selecting information for inclusion or exclusion is not straightforward or lacking in purpose or strategy. The rhetorical compulsion of the court report locates its author firmly within the drama.

If the drama of the case requires an explainer, albeit an 'engaged' explainer, it needs also an excuser, the defending lawyer, someone who, in the course of a long career, will make more feeble excuses for more criminals than will any social worker. The distinction between excuser and explainer is important. The competent 'excuser' is insulated against opprobrium from press, public or judiciary by the instructional nature of the client relationship. He or she is rightly regarded as an articulate mouthpiece for the client's views who, though stopping short of deception, doubtless takes most of what has to be said with a liberal pinch of salt. Occasionally, indeed, excusers communicate a certain scepticism by such distancing strategies as gesture, tone and terminology, strategies intended to be decoded by the court but not the client: their role in the drama is secure precisely because everybody knows it to be a piece of sanctioned deception which ironically legitimates the very process in which it is (but only formally) a dissenting element.

The 'explainer' on the other hand has a different and more disturbing role which involves both uttering the explanation and believing it: each explanation, therefore, contains an embryonic theory of human behaviour. There is about this an unavoidable politicality: while the explainer has the capacity to reassure, to complete the jigsaw picture, to make sense of the otherwise incomprehensible, the capacity is also there to challenge and disturb, to raise issues of moment which fall outside the agreed script of the proceedings. For this reason the explanation may be both more persuasive and more threatening than the excuse. Depending on the form of explanation chosen it can shift the discourse – about crime, parenting or human suffering – from the agreed, comfortable and individualised notions containable within that social formation of which the court is such an essential part to a framework whose logical conclusion is to challenge the legitimacy of the court itself.

The excuser, whose overt function it is to challenge, disturb, fight, paradoxically does none of these things except within the strict confines of the formulaic, the court ritual. It is no surprise that the court room is such a popular *locus* of popular fiction, a mode of asserting and reasserting that good will out, that the world is as it should be. The explainer's role, however, contains what MacIntyre calls a 'moral incommensurability' (MacIntyre 1981: 68) between the conflicting urges to speak the particular and possibly challenging version of the 'truth' affirmed by professional value, 'theory' and socialisation and to speed the process of the trial itself by routinising, making the 'explanation' of the 'case' explicable and conventional. We shall see in Chapter 4 an interesting and unusual example of just how a moral incommensurability between two scripts, based, respectively, on 'rights' and 'utility', plays itself out when a social worker departs – dramatically – from his script.

This, however, is an extreme case and the experts do not normally offer such radical interpretations. That they do not indicates how restricted is their scope to translate any unconventional analysis into practical form: the range of possible outcomes is extremely limited. The question of whether the miscreant is an Oliver to be rescued or a Dracula to be disposed of is not primarily resolved by theoretical means but by strategic decisions based on factors which include occupational socialisation, agency policy, a prediction of what the court will want, available resources, a strong commitment to one's own professional survival and the received wisdom of the office tea room. Given this combination of factors a fairly conformist explanation is obviously probable.

Any interest on the part of the social professionals, therefore, in transcending the stereotype, in engaging with the phenomenology of the individual psyche, is daily mediated by a range of pressures – some material, some imagined – and the outcome is typically a routinisation which can itself be defended as 'just'. Still, however, there are choices, and if the professionals have, since their more strident days of the 1970s, had their claws removed as they have secured a firmer *locus* in the court room, the choices still have an obvious and immediate impact on the juvenile. For the routinisation which is so 'just' relates not primarily to any 'real' or 'essential' characteristic of the youngster but to the mode of depiction. In the social world we do not move in some post-Humean empiricist manner from cause to effect – from expert and objective analysis to confident outcome, from assessment to disposal (Wicker 1975: 18–19): on the contrary, the desired or expected mode of disposal influences the materials selected for assessment. It is in this sense that the court report becomes a strategic and rhetorical document, for while it does (of course) move conventionally from premiss to conclusion, it simultaneously couches its premisses in such a way as to make the desired outcome probable, if not inevitable.

CONCLUSION

Our understanding of children and their needs and behaviour, families, the role of the experts and the state which employs them is simplified and therefore limited. This chapter has sought to explore, historically and by contemporary analysis, some of the ways in which we collectively pursue this understanding. We have done so using the concepts, which seem to us both prevalent and apt, of narrative and drama. The events which revolve round juvenile delinquency are 'dramatic', the experts are part of that 'drama', they make sense of this experience by 'telling stories'. To tell stories is not, however, to abandon 'reality' for the make-believe world of fiction, nor is the employment of narrative, tale and drama as a conceptual framework to trivialise or academicise the choices or minimise the suffering of 'real' people. The marginalisation of narrative is itself a cultural act (see, for example, Tambling 1991), and the division of the world into 'real' and 'fictional' ignores the extent to which we draw on both for our day-to-day interpretations:

> narrative is present in myth, legend, fables, tales, short stories, epics, history, tragedy, *drame* [suspense drama], comedy, pantomime, paintings . . . stained glass windows, movies, local news, conversation. Moreover, in this infinite variety of forms, it is present at all times, in all places, in all societies; indeed narrative starts with the very history of mankind; there is not, there has never been anywhere, any people without narrative . . . . Like life itself, it is there, international, trans-historical, transcultural.
>
> (Barthes 1975: 237)

Our concern in this book is to take as a case study a point of decision where the choice seems clear – between locking up a child and not – and to examine why that choice is in truth anything but clear. As we have seen, secure accommodation is as ambiguous a disposal as the behaviour and experiences of the child under consideration are ambiguous, and though it is now rare for social workers to recommend courts to commit a youngster to penal custody, the same restraint does not exist with secure accommodation. We do not quite agree with those who say that this is hypocrisy or self-deception, the distinction between secure accommodation and prison false, for patently it is a 'real' distinction not only in the eyes of the social workers but in terms of policy and practice within the units themselves.

Yet the paradox remains: secure accommodation is a custodial provision available to and managed by a profession which has set its stall against custodial provisions. Criteria for its use exist and the social workers have to persuade the court that they apply in a given case. It is while engaging in this strategic pursuit that the social workers choose their story, deciding whether the child is, for the time being at least, devil, mucky angel, neither or both. How and why this situation has come about, how and why secure accommodation is splitting at the seams, with social workers demanding more of it while opposing custody and asserting the importance of 'self-determination', are questions to be addressed in this book. Something rather complicated appears to be going on.

Part II

Secure accommodation

Some themes and issues from an empirical study

4 Talking to the experts

> Decisions . . . are ultimately made by a court. But this is only the final point of the process of decision-making.
>
> (Hilgendorf 1981: 1)

> We don't treat children any differently from children in the open unit except that they can't get out.
>
> (Interviewee)

SECURE ACCOMMODATION: SOME BACKGROUND ISSUES

In Chapter 1 we outlined the background to the concerns which prompted the study discussed in this chapter, portraying secure accommodation as a strategy in search of a policy, an historically explicable and probably necessary attempt to contain a problem with no solution. Secure accommodation grew exponentially throughout the 1970s, but in an uncoordinated way: the concomitance during this decade of the existence of secure accommodation itself and of the belief that disturbed or disturbing youngsters could be effectively 'treated' in the face of their implacable rejection of the best efforts of the caring professionals (we might indeed say the virtual necessity of secure accommodation in the light of this belief) led to the rapid designation of new categories of children to be committed to secure accommodation, that their possibly unrecognised needs or interests might the better be met.

In the 1970s the containment of delinquents in penal establishments was not especially politically contentious, and the fact that the cost of the containment was met by central government created a financial incentive for local authorities to encourage it. Certainly there was a strong view, within the units themselves and in DHSS, that the unsatisfactory state of the prisons should not be used to justify transferring criminal youngsters to the care system; and the therapeutic orientation of local authority units rested uneasily with the remand function: not only were remanded youngsters not selected for therapy, but to offer it might prejudice their trial.

By the end of the 1970s, however, a significant shift in both economic and political preoccupations had occurred, and a new professional interest in children's rights emerged. This was reflected in a more sceptical approach to the twin assumptions that social workers were the best people to take decisions about needs and interests and that the benefits of secure accommodation itself were uncontestable.

Most significantly, the concept of 'rights' was entering the vocabulary of child care. American literature was identifying 'treatment' as theoretically and politically suspect (American Friends Service Committee 1971; Von Hirsch 1976); and this, together with the increasing influence of the legal lobby on the newly elected government of 1979, the impact on government of the *X* v. *The United Kingdom* judgment in 1981, the campaigning work of the Children's Legal Centre, the existence of well-coordinated pressure groups supported from within DHSS, the impact of two critical studies (Millham *et al.* 1978; Cawson and Martell 1979) and government's suspicion of executive decision making and resistance to large-scale capital projects combined to create an irresistible force for change.

These changes were reflected in the pattern of DHSS capital expenditure for secure units. Successive Departmental triennial reports indicate a steady upward trajectory from the mid-1970s onwards, peaking at £2 million in 1980/81, falling somewhat (to £1,748,000) the following year, and collapsing to £525,000 in 1982/83. These trends mirrored the numbers of secure places available: 205 in 1975/76, rising to almost 500 in 1981/82 but falling to 382 in 1984. A number of authorities closed their secure units in the early 1980s, partly in the belief that the rapid expansion of the 1970s had led to over-provision, and partly because they did not wish to meet the improved standards now required for inspectorial approval and hence a DHSS licence. All these figures, of course, fell far short of the projections of need made in the mid-1970s (House of Commons 1975: para. 72).

Alongside these changes had occurred some significant shifts in the child population of secure units. The increasing scepticism about prisons shared by many politicians, civil servants, academics and professionals from the late 1970s led to pressure to transfer children in adult prisons to secure units, a trend which, by the mid-1980s, was widely endorsed by the local authorities themselves. The comments of a number of interviewees about 'their' children to whom 'they' had a responsibility were made in the light of strongly negative views of prison: several used phrases such as 'prison's the end of the road' and 'once they've gone there we've lost them', and seemed concerned to save 'their' children from an experience whose destructiveness would have consequences with which they, as the care authority, would later have to deal anyway.[1]

As a result of these changes, the *locus* of secure accommodation in the child-care system shifted: the proportion of children in secure accommodation in care under the civil jurisdiction fell steadily during the 1980s while the proportion of remandees increased. At the same time the number of youngsters in secure accommodation not as a result of a 21A authorisation but under the provisions of the Children and Young Persons Act 1933, section 53(2), was also rising. This section provided for the detention for up to a specified period (there being provision for executive release on licence) of children and young persons found to have committed manslaughter, attempted murder or wounding with intent to do grievous bodily harm. For many years the provision was hardly used, but the Criminal Justice Act 1961 extended its scope to include juveniles who had committed an offence punishable in the case of an adult by fourteen years' imprisonment.[2] As a result, juvenile burglars and rapists who would previously have been dealt with custodially came to be caught in the 53(2) net, and the section was, probably unintentionally, transformed from a last-ditch social defence into a tariff sentence. Henceforward any increase in courts' sentencing powers in respect of adults (by making more offences imprisonable by fourteen-year terms) would have a knock-on effect on juveniles' eligibility for 53(2) (Godsland and Fielding 1985), and thereby on the population of secure units. While 53(2) is still not commonly used, and although some 53(2) children are held in mental hospitals and youth treatment centres, the effect on secure accommodation is cumulative, with disproportionate pressure on beds being exerted by this numerically small but proportionately increasing group of long-term residents.

THE RESEARCH OUTLINED

The Leicester University research was commissioned by DHSS to study the impact on the use of secure accommodation of the new requirement that local authorities obtain an authorisation from a juvenile court before holding children in secure accommodation for more than 72 hours in any 28-day period. The study began two years after the change was implemented, and this, combined with the fact that no prior national statistics on the use of secure accommodation existed, prevented us from undertaking a 'before–after' study. For three main reasons, however, it is unlikely that such a study would have been satisfactory.

First, the widespread availability of draft legislation meant that most authorities had been developing policies consistent with it for over a year prior to implementation. Secondly (a significant finding in its own right), insufficient pre-implementation departmental policy documents existed to enable us to mount an effective comparison. Thirdly, we learned that any assumption that a simple causal relation existed between the introduction of section 21A and the policies of local authorities would have been incorrect. As we have already argued theoretically, legislative change relatively seldom simply 'causes' changes in social actions: the processes of law making characteristically reflect the very changes to be enforced by new legislation, emerging when an 'incoherence in the arrangements of the society' presses convincingly for remedy (Oakeshott 1962: 124). While it would be incorrect to dismiss the creative and generative functions of law, they coexist with the reflective purpose of codifying and legitimating changing forms of social behaviour.

The research sought to answer three questions:

1 How do local authorities act in the light of 21A?
2 What problems do they encounter?
3 Does the system (in particular the judicial review) act in the best interests of the child?

These questions were to be answered in four intersecting studies: a *background study* involving interviews with key individuals involved in national debates about secure accommodation; a *national policy survey* of all local authorities; a *criteria study* of the workings of a sub-sample of eleven authorities, involving both a content analysis of the files of all children from the authority who had been in secure accommodation since the introduction of 21A and interviews with the children in secure accommodation at the time of our visit and with their key decision makers; and an *observational study* of juvenile courts hearing applications for secure accommodation authorisations.

The *background study* explored the politics of secure accommodation and helped us formulate questions for the later parts of the study. It involved exploratory interviews with academics, researchers, managers, solicitors, secure unit practitioners, civil servants, social reformers and politicians representing a wide variety of positions in the secure accommodation debate, and was undertaken successfully. The *national policy survey*, however, in which a closed questionnaire was to be administered to all local authorities, was abandoned shortly after the research began, for pilot interviews with senior social services personnel reinforced our growing suspicion that the ambiguities and complexities already identified would be concealed by survey methodology (for a fuller discussion on policy analysis methodology see Hardiker *et al.* 1991: 53–64).

For example, we were interested in the relation between the frequency of secure accommodation applications and the organisational level at which the decision to make an application could be made. It quickly became clear that this level varied remarkably, and since the main reason for creating a narrow decision filter was to ration usage it was important to test whether this strategy was effective. As one Deputy Director put it:

> There was a need to reduce expenditure on out-of-county placements, and the decision-making on whether or not a child could be placed out of county for any purpose had been placed with the Deputy Director. So I inherited the agency placements budget and obviously secure accommodation placements tended to be the most expensive, and I inherited that too.

When pilot interviews probed this, however, a distinction emerged between formal and effective decision making. So Agency A, which claimed the decision was made at Assistant Director level, did indeed require the Assistant Director's signature, but only to rubber-stamp a 'decision' made at a lower level. In Agency B, however, staff members seeking approval were interrogated by a Principal Officer and asked to produce 'alternative packages' to secure accommodation. Hence, while the formal decision was made at a higher level in Agency A, the effective decision was made at a lower level than in Agency B.

Clearly therefore, it would be impossible to discover the level of decision making within agencies without more detailed organisational analysis. Surveys were accordingly replaced by a *policy study* of fifty local authorities, selected on a stratified basis to ensure representativeness in relation to four variables: the possession or not of a secure unit; high, medium and low usage of secure accommodation as a proportion of children in care; geographical location; and population size. Each area was visited once and a taped interview conducted with the manager with decision-making responsibility for secure accommodation. This change in method enabled us to probe further, identifying aspects of the complex relation between policy and practice. Since the interview was preceded by a list of nineteen prior notice questions, the interview took place, theoretically at least, with any statistical information we required having been produced and digested by the interviewee.

The *criteria study*, which involved a sub-sample of eleven authorities, fell into two parts: a retrospective analysis of file data on all youngsters admitted to secure accommodation in the authority since the legislative change in May 1983, and a decision-tracing exercise in respect of children currently in secure accommodation, involving interviews both with the children themselves and with key professionals. Though it had originally been intended to undertake a similar decision-tracing exercise in the retrospective study to complement the content analysis, inadequacies of file data and high levels of staff mobility joined forces with our own resource limitations to thwart this intention.

The *court observations* sought to identify the relationship between the formal expectation that courts would protect children's rights against the local authorities and what in fact occurred. Organising the observations proved difficult both because of the infrequency with which applications were made and the lack of notice available in what transpired to be the crucial first applications. Whereas there was little difficulty in arranging to observe renewal applications, the majority of these were rubber-stamping exercises. This, though an important finding in its own right, meant that observations were seldom necessary.

First applications were frequently late additions to the lists, and because they were so few in number not only was it difficult to observe sufficient hearings in a realistic time-scale, but officials in the clerks' department were only variably successful at remembering to notify us. We concentrated on five 'high usage' courts where we might reasonably have expected perhaps one new application most weeks; we then hired and trained suitable local people (research students or retired court personnel) to attend court at short notice and complete a schedule which combined hard and impressionistic data.

Obvious frustrations are inherent in this strategy, and we failed to meet our target of observing eighty hearings. The thirty-seven we did observe, however, yielded such consistent data that we are satisfied that our findings fairly represent the work of the courts which make the majority of authorisations.

THE POLICY STUDY

In this chapter we focus primarily on the policy study, which entailed visiting fifty agencies to interview the manager responsible for approving applications for secure accommodation authorisations. To give a 'view from the sharp end', however, we also report those parts of the interviews with professionals undertaken in the criteria study which raise general issues. Front-line workers experience most directly the consequences of the agency's secure accommodation policies: flexible policies give them the onerous responsibility of making judgements in difficult cases; rigid policies prevent them using secure accommodation to contain seemingly insoluble problems.

In the policy study we interviewed personnel from Directors of Social Services to middle managers with an assortment of job titles and duties; though most had a 'child-care' brief, not all had control of a budget. On a number of occasions we found on arriving that we were meeting not only the individual with whom we had made the appointment but another staff member, normally junior to the intended interviewee, who was typically introduced as having day-to-day responsibility for secure accommodation issues and being more in touch with the 'nuts and bolts'. This person, whose role appeared to be either to provide moral support for an anxious superior or to constitute an admiring audience (or perhaps both), normally played only a minor part in the interview. On one occasion we were asked to attend a secure unit itself, where we met eight members of staff, including unit workers and a visiting psychiatrist.

Interviews were conducted on the basis of a guided schedule and prior notice questions. We do not report here detailed (but now outdated) information about the extent of provision, finance, occupancy and referral rates and so on, drawing on it only to make a number of more general and relevant observations. The managers to whom we spoke were narrators. As we have seen, however, there are narrators and narrators: some are reliable, some unreliable; some are omniscient, some ignorant of key factors; some are dispassionate and detached from the events of the *histoire* while others are centrally involved in the action (for a classic consideration of these issues, see Booth 1961). We then discuss three topics which emerged as particularly significant means of highlighting matters which concern us here: the management of the '72-hour rule', the decision to apply for an authorisation and interviewees' opinions of the nature and character of DHSS inspections of secure units. In these three areas the local authority is, respectively, decision maker, applicant and inspected, three distinct roles which, together, give us a rounded picture of secure accommodation and how it fits into the structures of the social services department.[3]

In the following sections we both provide information about our subject and discuss the manner in which it was presented to us: our data are both *histoire* and narrative. When we are told something we form a judgement not only about the events but about the narrator, whose function is one of mediacy (Stanzel 1984) between *histoire* and reader, shaping as well as reporting the *histoire* itself. Inevitably, therefore, we ask such questions as 'Why is this person telling me this?', 'Is this person truthful?', 'Is this person dependable or deceived by others?'. This process is basic to oral communication, though more problematic with written materials because the reader is unable to interpret the multi-layered forms of non-verbal communication familiar to social psychologists. This, of course, is part of the reason why a number of theorists from Socrates onwards mistrust writing and relegate it to a position inferior to orality (Derrida 1976: ch. 1).[4]

The men (and, less often, women) whom we interviewed, then, told us their stories. Some were eloquent, some stumbling and relatively inarticulate. Some glanced periodically at the tape recorder, and one referred apprehensively to everything 'going down on acetate'. Some played to a fine art the role of organisational representative, others dropped this role, playing instead the wise insider, the critic of agency or court. Several contrasted the practices of their own agencies favourably with those of neighbouring agencies or former employers. Some, in a manner which reminded us that in narrative theory the role of the narratee, and in particular the narrator's perception of it, is crucial too (Prince 1982), saw us as conduits to DHSS and delivered variably lengthy sets of policy proposals directly to our tape recorder, with which they sometimes established a rapport evidenced by prolonged and empathic eye contact.

Occasionally, when visiting contiguous departments, we heard both sides of the same inter-agency conflict, different narrations of the same *histoire*. For example, Agency C had invested considerable resources in a secure unit partly on the basis of a commitment from neighbouring Agency D, which, in return for contractually agreed payments, received specified usage rights. Agency D withdrew from this commitment at short notice, explaining this to us in terms which indicated that its progressive child-care policies, which involved providing more variegated forms of care, were being impeded by disproportionate expenditure on the neighbouring secure unit. In these terms Agency D's decision to withdraw was an heroic rejection of an outmoded form of treatment, in future to be used only *in extremis*. To Agency C, however, Agency D had 'ratted' by reneging on a contract, thereby, since the premises were insufficiently versatile to be converted for other uses, leaving it with a 'great white elephant', a heavy deficit on the child-care budget and worries about (as it then was) rate capping.

Agency C's response to this problem was to engage in aggressively marketing the unit to other authorities, successfully selling beds to a wider range of customers. Agency C, therefore, told us a tale in which, though it was the innocent victim of Agency D's perfidy, it yet rose again and proceeded to ultimate triumph. This stood in stark contrast to the Agency D version in which *it* was the hero, bravely casting aside the outmoded practices of a bygone era, doing the best for its children in the face of hostility and contumely.

We cannot, of course, determine who is the victim, who the villain, for neither of these 'simple tales' encompasses, even expresses, the complexity of the conflict. How, as Alasdair MacIntyre asks, do we weigh conflicting moral principles – here the principle of adherence to a contract against that of progressive and humane policy development – in a society which lacks the very forms of authority which would guide us inexorably to elevate one over the other?

> we have all too many disparate and rival moral concepts, in this case rival and disparate concepts of justice, and . . . the moral resources of the culture allow us no way of settling the issue between them rationally. Moral philosophy, as it is dominantly understood, reflects the debates and disagreements of the culture so faithfully that its controversies turn out to be unsettlable in just the way that the political and moral debates themselves are.
>
> (MacIntyre 1981: 235)

THE INTERVIEWS: SOME TOPICS AND THEMES

Autonomy retained: the 72-hour rule

The notion that restrictions on local authorities' use of secure accommodation should not preclude emergency action has been relatively uncontroversial. Under the '72-hour rule' local authorities may contain youngsters for up to three days in any 28-day period without recourse to the courts. Such an arrangement was in fact advocated in an influential report (Children's Legal Centre 1982: 28), albeit with more restrictions on its implementation than have been introduced: whereas the Children's Legal Centre argued that authorisations of 24–72 hours should be made by a member of staff of at least Principal Officer level this was not translated into regulation, presumably reflecting central government sensibility to intervening in the internal decision making of a local government department.

Not surprisingly, given the ambiguity which we have stressed throughout, during the background study we were several times told of widely varying practices in relation to the 72-hour rule. Some authorities were said to use it as a miniature of authorised secure accommodation itself, some for repeated but short 'cooling-off periods' for troublesome children, some as an emergency protective measure while a case was being prepared for court, while some, apparently, did not use it at all.

In 72-hour cases local authorities are decision makers, not supplicants; arguably therefore, the operation of such cases accurately represents the agency's 'true' picture of secure accommodation. It would be difficult, after all, for a respondent to confess to using secure accommodation in 'short bursts' as a controlling device while arguing that it was also a 'last resort'. Similarly, we might look for the forms of policy which exist in the agency, not so much – or not only – for their content, but because the very existence of a document signals a certain seriousness and concern. More fundamentally, however, our respondents, like the narrators we have already discussed, may be variably involved in the drama of the cases. A detached narrator might maintain a clear conscience but at the cost of creating an insoluble problem further down the line by returning the problematic child to the very workers whose failure to deal with him provoked the initial pressure for secure accommodation. An involved narrator, on the other hand, might share the problem and not claim exclusive rights to the solution.

The spread of practices, we discovered, was not primarily a matter of 'professional ideology' or opinion: in fact, on this comfortably abstract plane significant points of rhetorical consonance emerged around factors deemed to constitute good child care – offering individual relationships, providing appropriate care and treatment, focusing on rehabilitation, enhancing self-worth and dignity. Of greater interest was the plethora of conflicting practices which emerged from these consensual abstractions. Fundamental differences permeated the structures of policy making within the agencies. We asked interviewees whether their authorities had policy documents on the 72-hour rule. One did not know; of the forty-nine who did twenty-seven said 'yes' and twenty-two 'no'. Forty respondents could tell us who in the authority was empowered to authorise containment, though in only sixteen cases was the expectation of the Children's Legal Centre met that the decision should be made at Principal Officer level or above. Few provider authorities knew how often the 72-hour rule was invoked and typically referred us to records kept at the local unit and not submitted to headquarters.

Whether or not a policy document on the 72-hour rule existed, thirty authorities claimed to restrict usage to 'emergencies' (however defined), several permitted holdings only as a prelude to court hearings, others made no restrictions. Though a few references to 'cooling-off periods' were made, no interviewee admitted permitting repeated usages to contain difficult youngsters. One interviewee objected to fettering colleagues' discretion; another pointed to the dangers of permitting movement between an open and a secure unit on the same premises on the ground that 'if they know there is a secure unit at the end of the run then they will not work as hard dealing with the children in open conditions because it seems a way out'; and a third asserted unambiguously that the principle of deprivation of liberty was the same whatever the length of the containment period:

> For the 72 hours we tend to take the same line: we're as stringent with the 72 as if we're going to court, because that's where you will eventually be going . . . you've got to be absolutely clear about that because that's where abuse can come in.

We were also interested in what thought had been given to managing, supporting and training staff. Here and elsewhere we were struck by the curious phenomenon that overlying the ambiguities about 'security' already discussed there is the dimension that unit staff too are 'in' secure accommodation, only slightly less subject to the power of the institution than the youngsters (for an interesting perspective on this see the interviews in Glouberman 1990). Typically, staff spend longer in the institution than children (only 4 per cent of those discharged in 1986 had been in secure accommodation more than 6 months) (DHSS 1986); they too are subject to instructions from above; many are closer in age to the youngsters than to their managers. The units manifest a form of 'security' which insulates staff as well as inmates from other influences. Staff typically work in very small units – many with fewer than ten beds – sometimes geographically removed from the main centres of population and professional activity. Many are untrained sub-professional employees, marginal to the main enterprise of their agency yet with the awesome duty of holding against their will some of the most difficult and disturbed of the agency's clientele:

> Staff in secure units could themselves be metaphorically locked in to that form of provision and cut off from the field of residential social work or child care. There were financial disincentives for teaching staff to leave for mainstream teaching jobs. Other categories of staff might not have an occupational identity outside their CHE [community home with education], and so be highly dependent on powerful heads. A high proportion were unqualified and their opportunities for professional or broader based training were more limited than those of other staff in residential care. Geographical isolation in some cases exacerbated their professional and managerial isolation.
>
> (Henkel 1991a: 130)

There was some acknowledgement of the training implications of restrictive usage policies for poorly paid, low-level inexperienced staff, and several respondents acknowledged that it was easy for senior managers to espouse liberal principles while leaving consequential issues to workers described in interchangeable metaphors as being at 'the sharp end' or 'the coal face'. Yet though some interviewees referred to the problems of unit staff (one Director deploring the 'disgraceful' salaries he was permitted to pay residential workers), none could produce a training strategy to help staff manage discretion, enhance their skills in, for example, behaviour management or conflict reduction, or integrate their units with those broader departmental child-care policies from which they seemed often to be far removed. One Principal Officer, asked about secure unit staff training, admitted:

> It's very *ad hoc*. . . nobody has ever made a proper assessment of their training needs. What we've done from time to time is respond to strange

> situations as they arose – for example on sexual issues when we had a number of girls in the unit who were very sophisticated prostitutes and knew more about it than the staff. Then the staff can join the large countywide training schemes . . . . They run their own things from time to time.

It is this final layer of the ambiguous and amorphous concept 'security' which lies behind the management of the '72-hour rule'. The Children's Legal Centre, as we have seen, argued that decisions about usage should be taken at senior management level. Not surprisingly, given the startling disparities in approach and usage which our study uncovered, we have sympathy for this view. Merely to raise the organisational level of decision making, however, is again to confuse cause and effect. The *minutiae* of law and policy are, in the day-to-day world of courts and governments, regularly subsumed by the exigency of immediate problem solving. If a child behaves so as to defy all available resources, it is pointless to operate a *withdrawal strategy* which debars the workers who have to manage children from placing them in secure accommodation because it is precisely to deal with such situations that secure accommodation is necessary. A better way to proceed is by a *supplementation strategy* of increasing resources, so that a higher proportion of difficult youngsters can be contained other than in security.

The almost inevitable consequence of seeking to restrict the use of secure accommodation by withdrawal alone is either to heighten danger to staff, other children and the child in question or to provoke an occupational deviance culminating in policy manipulation or more extreme and negative activities. One example of such action was the illicit form of secure accommodation known as 'pindown', developed between 1985 and 1991 in Staffordshire, involving the solitary confinement of difficult youngsters. The system, though 'unplanned', was, curiously, a secret to which almost everyone seemed party: 'It was a sudden response . . . we created things very quickly, names and things very quickly. I can't recollect any major plan of putting it together' (cited in Levy and Kahan 1991: 29).

If we are truly to understand the problems of secure accommodation it is pointless to restrict ourselves to explanations defining the actions of individuals as first causes, for, deplorable as these actions doubtless were, they were also the products of the kind of arrangements we have been describing. The pindown report comes close to recognising this, but fails to pursue the logic of its own analysis. This failure causes it to stumble into the conceptual confusion as well as linguistic infelicity of the 'double however' in this key passage:

> We would hope that the frank and explicit nature of the records and

> comments in the log book only represent a temporary aberration on their part. One cannot, *however,* erase the knowledge that the active life of Pindown was within a month of six years. We must, *however*, recognise that the residential staff were carrying out difficult work without being provided by their employers with adequate supervision, support, resources or even proper understanding in many cases of their task.
>
> (Italics added. Levy and Kahan 1991: 169)

To make this point is not to condone the actions of the workers but to stress that staff as well as residents are 'in' closed institutions. The institution develops its own *modus operandi*, and only, in what is only seemingly a paradox, by opening up the closed institution by involving the staff in a more integrated way with the day-to-day workings of the agencies will the problems currently permeating institutional life begin to be tackled.

To the Children's Legal Centre the issue is simple. Note in the following piece the singular form of 'use' (whereas it is surely clear that secure accommodation has many *uses*), the metaphorical use of 'shielded', and the word 'undisguised', implying a conspiracy to present one clearly encapsulated but shameful purpose in a visage which will be applauded by those who are to be deceived: therapy is the *alibi for* incarceration, not an aspect of it:

> The rapid growth in the use of secure accommodation in the child care system has been shielded from questioning partly [*sic*] by the development of euphemistic and confusing language: those who advocated its expansion in the sixties and early seventies were aware that public opinion might not tolerate the undisguised locking up of increasing numbers of young people.
>
> (Children's Legal Centre 1982: 4)

Though the Children's Legal Centre may be right to demand a centralisation of decision making under the 72-hour rule, this alone will solve one problem only at the expense of creating another. Reminiscent of Barthes's black soldier, encountered in Chapter 2, our view, *pace* the Children's Legal Centre, is that secure accommodation is neither a symbol of, nor an alibi for, the state's attitude towards children and families, but the very presence of it, the manifestation of an attitude affecting not the children and their families alone but also the staff charged with their management. There is neither clarity nor conspiracy at the heart of the matter: the state's attitude to children, even proletarian children, is patently not based simply on disguised repression, but is the product of an accumulation of traces which, though they take different forms, do indeed signify that a child is less than a citizen: to be punished and controlled, yes, but to be loved and, in Ariès's word, coddled too. Children in secure accommodation are characteristically both victims and threats (Eekelaar *et al.* 1982), the characters of classics not trash, posing problems which will not be solved routinely but which require mature, thoughtful and creative consideration.

The management of the 72-hour rule constitutes a further layer in the ambiguity with which children and childhood are viewed in contemporary Britain. The lack of opposition to the unfettered right of local authorities to hold children for up to 72 hours in any 28-day period signifies that even those 'reformers' concerned to protect children's rights believe the powers of the state over the child should be greater than those over the adult: there would after all be controversy if government sought to give the courts similar powers over mentally healthy adults. In the case of children, however, the triad of needs, rights and interests must be maintained *ensemble* if we are not to do damage. If, as seems indubitable, we cannot unproblematically apply simple rules to a particular case, what can we do beyond entrust the decision to experts who are themselves scrutinised by an outside body? The 72-hour rule is a part of this practical response, and the story told us by our respondents is of how the professionals, charged with containing an unanswerable problem, seek the best ways forward.

Applying for an authorisation: the bureau-professional decision

> [Director of Social Services] I had a call the other Saturday evening from a social worker about a kid who's in care to us. His father writes every so often to suggest I am dismissed for handling the case so badly. And this lad, he's 14 now, he absconds from everywhere he's put. We sent him to E Home (a community home with education 100 miles away) and he absconded from there and had been picked up by the police. The duty social worker spoke to E Home who wouldn't have him back; the police didn't want him in a cell and suggested that we put him in secure. I said I didn't want to lock him up and asked the fieldwork manager to have a word with E Home. He runs away but he's not a serious offender – more of a nuisance. And he phoned E Home and they agreed to take him back. And I think all that says is if the control rests high enough in the organisation you can ensure that people don't make easy decisions about children.

We have distinguished formal and effective decision making and shown that formal decision makers, though accountable for the decision, do not necessarily make it. This division of responsibility can reflect a range of relations within the organisation, from senior staff's trust or mistrust of more junior staff to a desire to 'hide' the decision making processes from others within the organisation or from external evaluators. In the case of secure accommodation, however, most interviewees argued for formal and effective decision making to lie in the same individual. This reflected the twin beliefs that centralisation would lead to *consistency* (for a helpful analogy with decision making in Scottish Children's Hearings, see Smith and May 1980) and *rationing* of a resource which was both professionally delicate and resource intensive: in short, it was deemed economically as well as professionally prudent to restrict decision making to specified staff members.

Decision making was characteristically located either in non-specialist senior staff of Assistant Director level or above or in specialist child-care staff, normally of Principal Officer level. Such staff might or might not have a devolved budget. Whatever their organisational level, all interviewees acted as gatekeepers, but we encountered both *strong* and *weak* gatekeepers. Consistently with our view that it is pointless simply to close down options for staff facing a difficult if not insoluble problem, we developed a preference for decisions to be taken by 'strong' gatekeepers who, rather than simply saying 'no', had expert knowledge of alternative resources, the capacity to determine what resources were needed in a particular case, who were of sufficient seniority to develop new resources in response to need, active enough in national child-care circles to be aware of what developments were taking place elsewhere, who had sufficient research skills to monitor and evaluate the facilities, and who had control of a budget from which payment for secure units or places was made.

We believe decisions about secure accommodation applications are best taken by staff with responsibility for managing and resourcing child-care policies generally and that the gatekeeper in question should have a direct continuing responsibility for the children: it is undesirable for that responsibility merely to be bounced back to the very staff for whom such children have already presented insoluble problems. This continuing responsibility is part of the character of strong gatekeepers, one of whom, who particularly impressed us, had achieved a demonstrable and significant downturn in the use of secure accommodation in a high crime London borough while preventing any unjustifiable expansion of community control.

It follows that we do not support the simple view that the higher in the organisation the decision is taken the better, and we found no evidence that this was overall a major factor in determining the level of applications made. Though we did encounter a small number of cases where seniority was crucial (and our epigraph is an example of this), staff at Assistant Director level and above were more likely to be weak gatekeepers, senior but not expert, operating a rationing device rather than offering consultation to junior colleagues who were in some cases in despair as to what to do. 'Weak' gatekeepers, whose strategy was simply 'to give the social worker a hard time' but not necessarily to advise on alternatives, appeared simply to be delaying the inevitable: the likely consequence of throwing a difficult child back on the existing resources of area team or open establishment was that further requests would follow and eventually the 'no' would become 'yes'.

We were especially interested in how respondents perceived the respective roles of local authority and juvenile court in influencing the process. It would be possible, for example, for the local authorities to take the *legalistic view* that responsibility for determination rested with the court, the duty of the local authority being simply to check that a case was winnable before proceeding to the application hearing. Alternatively, a local authority might exercise *professional judgement* about the desirability of holding a youngster in security or *financial judgement* based on such criteria as budgetary prioritisation or availability, value for money and the cost of transportation to distant units. It would be possible, therefore, for a youngster to pass through three decision filters to determine eligibility, suitability and justifiability.

The first of these approaches was very rare, though many interviewees expressed relief that, as at least one of them put it, 'the buck stops with the court'. Almost all respondents referred to secure accommodation as a 'last resort', and a number of authorities had a policy of using the 'least restrictive' alternative. Some respondents felt the criteria were too wide:

> The criteria do leave open a very wide variety of interpretations . . . . I'm always conscious that different people in different authorities are probably using quite different interpretations, and once or twice we've taken a stand where others might not have done.

Two extreme authorities were Authority F, whose practice was for the recommendations of junior staff to be rubber-stamped by the Assistant Director, and Authority G, which declined, for political reasons, to co-operate with the research, but whose published documentation we none the less analysed:

> On 21 December 1983, the Social Services Committee agreed that both of the following criteria must be satisfied if HQ staff are to be allowed to authorise a child's placement in secure accommodation.
>
> (i) that the child has exhibited a history of persistent violence, evidenced by *repeated conviction f*or actual bodily harm, grievous bodily harm, malicious wounding, attempted murder or robbery (or offences of a similar nature and gravity)

AND

(ii) that there is *positive evidence* that the situation cannot be contained in an open placement.

It will be seen that there are marked differences between the local authority's criteria and the statutory criteria. The Committee felt the statutory criteria lacked precision, particularly in view of the seriousness of the decision for which they are intended and the possible adverse effects which the placement might cause the child in the short and/or long term.

(Italics added)

Authority F, on the other hand, was one of two in the sample where respondents rejected in principle the idea that courts, not social workers, should determine the use of secure accommodation: its image of secure accommodation was of a refuge, closer to hospital than prison, a place where problems were solved, and security, therapy and professional care provided, and always in a child's best interests. There could scarcely be a starker contrast with the view of Authority G that secure accommodation was prison *tout court*, to be reserved for violent juvenile recidivists in respect of whom there had to be *separate* 'positive evidence' [*sic*] that open containment was impossible.

Though Authority F's position may appear quaint to people attuned to contemporary debates in juvenile justice and child care, it should not be dismissed out of hand. It was a dominant view in the 1970s and may for all we know become so again, for history did not end yesterday. One could certainly mount an argument that the child's social worker was best placed to make judgements about both needs and interests, and that for a quasi-judicial tribunal to determine the matter would be for the state, in protecting rights, to damage interests. That many children in secure accommodation would, if at large, make damaging, even fatal, decisions was expressed forcefully: 'A lot of our youngsters, had they not had the advantage of going into secure would clearly be dead by now. Many are on the verge of suicide.' Children self-evidently do not always know what is best for them, and if their judgement has not been fine-tuned by responsible parents must not the state help them learn? And where the nature of the damage done leads the child into self-destructive activities, is it not the duty of the state to keep the child 'secure' in order to help? One interviewee (not from Authority F) said:

Often the youngsters who come to us have had various sorts of problems in the family and we use groups, lots of different methods, to get them to actually look at the way they interact with other people, look at the

> way they deal with difficult feelings and maybe get them to learn different ways of dealing with feelings. Lots of the children have been involved in glue sniffing in an effort to rid themselves of the pain of rejection or the pain of losing a parent or whatever. Once they come to us we encourage them to talk about this pain, to express it, to not try and get rid of it by sticking your head in a bag of glue or whatever. . . . Then we can begin to look at how they can cope on the outside again.

While it would be easy for the policy maker to deplore these inter-authority variations, to lament the process of justice by geography which they demonstrate (and we would not distance ourselves from such strictures), to the social analyst the divergence is both interesting and important. Whereas Authority F does not really acknowledge that secure accommodation has a punitive dimension, that rights as well as needs and interests are at stake, in Authority G the opposite position holds. Neither extreme reflects the ambiguity fundamental to the set of roles secure accommodation must play in child-care policy. If Authority F's policy continues unchecked, there is serious danger of the numbers of children being held escalating to politically unacceptable levels at the expense of developing creative alternatives; in Authority G, which rejects the notion that secure accommodation provides any form of physical protection for the self-destructive child, the social workers will be left with impossible and dangerous problems. Indeed it is clear that assaults on staff are one reason for admissions to secure units:

> This boy assaulted a female member of staff at H Children's Home. It was a violent assault and staff refused to contain him any longer, so an urgent request was made to J Secure Unit for them to take him.

We think that any local authority would find this policy difficult to defend either as responsible authority or as employer. A therapeutically orientated interviewee observed:

> I think the criteria are so stringent that you think of a kid . . . who is a runner and a runner, who is in total turmoil, I think you've got to look at each individual case and form a professional judgement. There is an argument that if you could use that (secure accommodation) for a month and keep the kid safe, secure [*sic*], you have the opportunity to work with it, to start untangling the bits, but if you can't meet the criteria then there's very often a number of cases that go into different categories simply because the criteria are so stringent . . . . Some kids do escalate up the ladder and become part of the inner city's homeless, aimless, drifting population. Sometimes you need to confront kids and the only way you force this is by locking them up for a short spell, and that's impossible now because of the new Act.

Secure accommodation cannot situate itself where either Authority F or G would place it without falling prey to the tyranny of the either–or. To grant sovereignty to any one of our trinity of needs, rights and interests is to confuse the simple with the simplistic and to initiate a new set of problems to replace those which have been put to one side. Part of our problem with Lorraine Harding's 'value perspectives' was that they are only superficially in opposition: all of them have merit, all are part of our cultural reservoir, any or all can properly be drawn on to tackle a problem. So it is with the positions of Authorities F and G: if we wish to embrace both the rights with which Authority G is concerned and the needs and interests which preoccupy Authority F, each of these perspectives is a necessary but not sufficient component of the social totality.

The accumulation of conflicting historical traces governing our understanding of childhood, our ambivalence about the intervention of the state in the realms of the 'private' family, the impossibility of creating 'rules' to embrace all the complex, troubled and troublesome youngsters who find themselves in secure accommodation gravitate against equating secure accommodation with hospital *or* prison, and demand that we continue to situate it in that shifting territory somewhere between the two. It is with this uneasy, even unreachable, task that our various respondents were struggling, enunciating principles, yet, in the day-to-day world of cases, finding good reason to depart from them, forever trying to be, in the paradoxical but only seemingly contradictory words of one, 'firm but flexible'.

Social services and the DHSS

> Very thorough, very good. Depending on which inspectors come determines how valuable we find it and how clear is the actual guidance that we get . . . . One is a bit of a waffler and you don't get straight answers, others are plain talking . . . . We get a four page letter covering all aspects of the visit and making recommendations.
>
> (Interviewee)

In this third sub-section the local authorities are neither decision makers nor (with all the complexities contained in the notion) expert advisers to the court, but examinees, their task performance being under the scrutiny of government inspectors. The ambiguities described in the two previous sub-sections are by no means absent here either.

Secure units were, at the time of our study, licensed by the DHSS (now the Department of Health) on the basis of periodic inspections conducted by the regional social services inspectorate (or SSI; for a fuller account of which see Henkel 1991a: 131 ff.). SSI replaced the Social Work Advisory Service (SWAS) in 1985 as part of government's intention to develop quality control based on hard measurement techniques (Henkel 1991a, b). The inspectorate has not, however, always found it easy to accommodate both its inspectorial functions and its shared professional affiliation with the agencies. The problem has both a strategic dimension – managing role strain – and an epistemological one:

> [The Inspectorate] introduced the language of objective measurement, input, output and outcome into the evaluation of quality of care, alongside that of process and subjective experience. Underpinning these two approaches are radically different views about the nature of social action and about knowledge of the social world, one using the language of cause and effect and generalizable laws of behaviour, the other that of meaning and motivation and shared or conflicting norms and beliefs.
> (Henkel 1991b: 131)

This ambiguity permeated interviewees' attitudes to the inspectors. While most spoke warmly of individual inspectors, inspection reports were widely regarded as consultative and advisory, not mandatory. A number of interviewees accordingly argued that though recommendations were to be taken seriously they were not necessarily to be implemented in full: inspectors did not, claimed one respondent, fully understand the complexity of the matter, and their reports were affected by the ambiguity surrounding secure accommodation. Presumably, if the purpose of secure accommodation is unclear, inspecting it cannot be straightforward, and the status of inspections must accordingly be diminished:

> Generally yes, they are helpful. I put a slight qualification in there because as local authorities we feel the DHSS are finding it very difficult to pin down at various times exactly what it is that is appropriate or not appropriate for a secure unit.

Inspections took place largely within the professional discourse of the inspected, and several respondents gave instances of collusions with inspectors designed to solve resource, policy or practical problems in a mutually desirable way. Henkel's study also demonstrated how inspections could become ammunition in the internal disputes which they inevitably highlighted; though painful and embarrassing, this could lead to future improvements:

> The last inspection at K Home was a shambles. Staff had made no real preparation. Indeed, the managers at K Home do not manage and he [senior manager] had found it hard to intervene. . . . The problem was one of power and long-standing resistance to interference on the part of

K Home. It was not just a question of inadequate support for staff, but also that the institution was being run to suit the interests of senior staff rather than children.

For example, some authorities used inspectors' comments on such aspects of the relationship between the physical environment and the quality of child care (Blumenthal 1985) as the state of repair of the buildings, or the absence of mirrors, to raise issues about the quality of care. In one inspection, holes in bedroom walls had been criticised, and senior managers had used this to challenge the view of unit staff that this was a matter of poor maintenance by the department, arguing instead that it demonstrated lack of care for the children. Similarly, an authority where there were serious disagreements between senior managers and heads of homes about body searches used inspectors' views to force a change in procedures. Another authority made approving reference to exploiting inspections to persuade the social services committee to reallocate resources. In all these cases we see instances of what we shall, in Chapter 5, term the power of the powerless – the capacity of subordinates in a relationship to manoeuvre an ostensibly disadvantageous situation to their advantage.

Government's intentions, in changing the culture as well as the name of the former SWAS, might be thought, therefore, to have been only partially successful. On the other hand, the view was put to us that inspections could only be effective if the inspectors obtained the cooperation from the inspected which derives from this shared affiliation. Though SSI has, since our fieldwork was conducted, further sharpened its quantitative measurement techniques (Henkel 1991b), it is still telling, if not exactly the same story as the inspected, then certainly one entirely recognisable by them.

The strengths of the inspections are also arguably their weakness. Inspectors can operate within the discourse of liberal professional values and, within that paradigm, comment on how particular units work. This increases the cooperation of the agencies but transforms the concept 'inspection' from a sceptical and dispassionate enquiry into an internal review: the inspection becomes a strategically negotiated, not an imposed, reality. In Saussure's terms this enables the SSI to interrogate the *parole* only, leaving the *langue* – the ordering of the relationships of which secure accommodation is a part – largely untouched.

TALKING TO THE PROFESSIONALS: SOME ISSUES AND DILEMMAS

As well as meeting the managers, we interviewed a range of lower-level professional staff who, in the course of discussing 'cases', raised many more general points. 'Sharp end' residential work involves containing the ambiguities we have been discussing, delicately managing needs, rights and interests from a position which locates the workers too as 'in' secure accommodation. Physically, numerically and professionally marginal to the main enterprise, unit workers operate a resource which, although it has the agency's imprimatur, the agency avoids using whenever possible. Theirs is the thankless task of dealing with the failures of more prestigious, better qualified and paid fieldwork staff while working in a setting which has many of the trappings of a black hole. Secure accommodation, after all, physically removes problem children from situations of higher visibility and politicality, enabling not only the child, in the words of one worker, to 'settle down into a routine' and, in those of another, to be 'stabilised', but the outside world to continue in reasonably ordered manner. This perception was shared by both field- and residential workers. One fieldworker described secure accommodation as: 'a nothingness . . . he just languishes in there, thinking this is OK because I don't have to think about anything [*sic*]'. Another said: 'In secure you can never really know how they're progressing until they come out, because it's such an unreal world.'

There is, in two distinct senses, something *unthinkable* about secure accommodation. In the strong sense the predominance of the 'locking up' motif in contemporary debate has stripped away some of the benign justification for secure accommodation, so creating for staff a role which makes many of them feel akin to prosecutors, sentencers and turnkeys. In the weak sense, the marginality of the provision makes it difficult for fieldworkers to *think about*, envisage, encapsulate and plan long term for their charges in the manner prescribed by the Department of Health. Workers use secure accommodation as a 'something', a temporary solution to a problem, but a destination reached by broad compass not precise signpost. Indeed, secure accommodation is precisely a bureau-professional manifestation of 'something': 'Something clearly had to happen and given that his behaviour wasn't improving anyway, and that the threats and violence were continuing, we had to start looking at something.' For front-line staff, subject to agency policy but with little involvement in initiating or developing it, these ambiguities are transformed into practical problems which both circumscribe and define the nature of their work. Though frequently described to us as 'contradictions', not all of these problems are consistent with our definition of contradiction provided in Chapter 2. All of them do, however, present practice dilemmas, and it is thus that we designate them. Here we note seven such dilemmas.

First, secure accommodation wards off custody only by *becoming* custody, a coercive intervention whose main justification is the utilitarian one that it is there to prevent something worse happening, a logic which decrees that if prisons were not so awful there would be no need for secure accommodation. Secure accommodation both prevents and is a 'manifest disaster', made none the less so by the fact that to a number of the children to whom we spoke the distinction between secure accommodation and custody, so clear to many of the professionals, was rather more opaque. Some children preferred the one, some the other; some preferred neither, others could not tell the difference; for others again the matter was of less import than questions of locality and the feasibility of family visits.

Secondly, many social workers too believed 'locality' important, wishing there were more neighbourhood facilities of which they could make use, while simultaneously arguing against opening more units in the belief that this would simply expand the system, leading to the incarceration of more children.

Thirdly, and in relation to finance, where secure accommodation accounts were not earmarked they were typically part of the child-care budget. The more secure accommodation was used, the more necessary it was felt to be to provide alternatives, but the fewer resources were available to do so, the necessary resources having been drained by secure accommodation itself. *Fourthly*, however, and in a further twist, the characteristic solution to this problem was to 'sell' secure places to other authorities, thereby creating the very 'dis-location' for out-county children which our second dilemma presents as antithetical to reintegration.

Planning was universally deemed fundamental to good child care. Here, however, we encountered a *fifth* dilemma, for the 'unthinkable' nature of secure accommodation seemed to drive it outside the planning scope partly because planning and emergencies cannot coexist comfortably, and partly because, as one interviewee remarked, if planning time were available it should be used to find an alternative to security. Hence, no doubt, the puzzlement of the unit manager who told us that though he received many enquiries from all over the country, he was never asked about his therapeutic orientation, only whether he had a bed available.

Sixthly, while field- and residential social workers appeared reasonably optimistic about the longer-term future of 'their' youngsters, they found themselves seeking to increase independence in a situation which diminished personal autonomy. One told us that 'in secure, people don't have to face up and make choices'; another wanted a half-way house in his (therapeutically orientated) unit, and found the legislation 'too black and white':

> We are all clear where we would like to go. The issue at the moment is how could we achieve a second stage unit on campus which would have

> the same culture, the same staff group, but which would not be physically secure. . . it is sometimes difficult when you are in a situation where you know a child is willing and accepting of help offered but we know we can only continue to offer it if the order is renewed. In many cases it might be arguable that the child does not technically fulfil the criteria. We are very much aware that there is a moral dilemma but at the moment we do not have the option.

The *seventh* dilemma arises when children 'choose' to be in secure accommodation. It illustrates the different perspectives on secure accommodation held by residential and field staff. To residential staff the challenge was to create and sustain precisely the kind of sensitive, caring and individualised facility in which children could flourish and in which, given the depressing circumstances from which most of them had emerged, they would, perfectly rationally, wish to stay. To fieldworkers, however, 'institutionalisation' was a powerful concept, and though they might also profess themselves committed to the equally problematic concept 'self-determination', so unthinkable was it to them that anyone would voluntarily go into secure accommodation that to do so was deemed symptomatic of institutionalisation itself, a therapeutic false consciousness exempting the professional from the obligation to take heed. Few workers saw their job as responding to the expressed wishes of their consumers. One girl had asked her social worker to seek a renewal:

> She said she felt safe in there: nobody was trying to get at her and there was no way she could abscond, and she did have more regular access to her father . . . . But we pointed out that that was not the reason for a secure unit. She would have to go back into the open unit and we would have to see how things went on.

In an ironic reversal of the orthodox view, one of our girl interviewees was to tell us that when she was moved from the secure unit to the open unit on the same site, her quality of life was so diminished that she regarded the move as punishment. For the boy in the following extract too, the ambiguity of secure accommodation remains a mystery:

Q What's it like here?
A I like it.
Q Doesn't it strike you as odd that you commit an offence and they lock you up in a nice place? Why do you think they do that?
A (*Laughs*) That's a question I've been asking myself, and I haven't been able to answer it.

He is, as will by now be apparent, not alone in his confusion.

CONCLUSION

In this chapter the professionals have had their say, and our theme of ambiguity may now have more flesh. The wording and implementation of legislation, the attitudes of professionals towards it, the relations between agencies and DHSS are all ambiguous. Even at a level of physical structure secure accommodation is not a 'thing' but a range of disparate institutions having in common only the possession of a licence and the turning of a key. The differences between, on the one hand, large, well-equipped, specialist units geared to meeting the needs of long-stay youngsters and, on the other, tiny holding establishments in the middle of the countryside are vast. Yet the chaos of allocation means that it is often chance where a youngster is sent: a confluence of body, bed and criteria is, as one respondent decisively told us, the prerequisite for a placement.

The ambiguity has particular implications for 'sharp-end' workers for whom these matters are anything but abstract, and manifests itself in a variety of dilemmas which determine the nature of the work itself and the relationship between child and worker. These dilemmas are not, however, simple confusions to be swept away by rewording legislation, rewriting regulations or issuing firmer briefs to the inspectorate, but a reflection of the nature of the job and the roles being enacted. The operation of the 72-hour rule, for example, reflects the beliefs, values, management style and alternative facilities of different departments as well, no doubt, as other more delicate factors defying detection in a single interview but turning on departmental micropolitics – the reputations of unit staff, strategic calculations, financial considerations, petty jealousies. In our study of decision making Authorities F and G were ideal type agencies, tailor-made to demonstrate ambiguity in action, seemingly impossible poles of the hospital–prison axis. As we travelled the country, however, yet a further layer of ambiguity became apparent to us, for we repeatedly received whispered confidences that in Authority G in particular things were not really like that, but were merely presented thus to placate an interventive committee. Such unsolicited rumours, innuendo and gossip, travelling like wildfire through this closed world in which we were temporary visitors, hint at the impossibility of attaining clarity and openness even in a corner of that world where things appeared simple and straightforward.

The most reliable predictor of high usage of secure accommodation was whether an agency was a 'provider' authority. No other variables – location of decision making, crime rate, size of care population, demography – gave us factors distinguishing high, medium and low users. We conclude, therefore, *either* that the mere existence of secure accommodation provokes its usage *or* that the pressures which led to a unit's construction in the first place continue to influence that usage. Managers' accounts certainly suggested that for an agency to sustain a secure unit was to give a cautious imprimatur to its use; and unit availability obviously eases any administrative problems surrounding admission. If application rates are currently depressed by shortage of places and consequential administrative inconvenience, and there is a widespread belief among the professionals that this is so, any disruption to the supply–demand balance by making available additional places must logically provoke increased usage. There must, therefore, for better or worse, be the likelihood of a repetition of the phenomenon of the expansionist 1970s when 'the boys in the units at present are less problematic than they have ever been' (Millham *et al.* 1978: 46).

This point is crucial. We argued in Chapter 2 that it is analytically incorrect to transfer the causal relations of the pure scientist's laboratory to the social world. Only in the anthropomorphic world of children's literature does the litmus paper strike back at the alkaline solution, protesting vociferously at the injustice of being turned blue, and, in taking active steps to avoid repetition, causing the said solution to reconsider its strategies. In the social world every cause results from something else, every result causes the next reaction. The logical and empirical impossibility of providing an unambiguous operational definition of the child who should, as opposed to the child who should not, enter secure accommodation[5] means that we must proceed by different means. In the social world measures of 'need' are not absolute but the products of the same social totality from which emerges the response to those 'needs'. If the 'response' is to make available more and better social provisions we must expect to witness a lowering of the threshold of the 'need' it is to meet (Harris 1990). Paradoxically, therefore, resources 'create' needs as much as needs 'cause' resources to be made available. Foucault's celebrated and subtle comment about prisons applies here too: 'although legal punishment is carried out in order to punish offences, one might say that the definition of offences and their prosecution are carried out in turn in order to maintain the punitive mechanisms and their functions' (Foucault 1977: 24). Nevertheless, the fact that the ambiguity of *between* hospital and prison or *thereabouts* lies at the heart of our problem should not lead us to believe ourselves helpless in the face of paradox and contradiction. As we have proceeded we have indeed made some suggestions and implied others. Here we mention just one, which is fundamental to much of this book. Like the Children's Legal Centre, we believe that the use of the 72-hour rule needs re-examining, if only because it seems impossible, as several interviewees told us, to divorce it from decisions about applying for authorisations. We have stressed, however, that it is insufficient to close down options, operating a withdrawal (as opposed to supplementation) strategy. The urgent problems presented by a difficult child cannot just be left, for they are unlikely to disappear. The supplementation, not only of facilities but of staff skill and support, is therefore necessary, but supplementation in a manner which avoids the 'net widening' effect stressed by social control theorists (Cohen 1985; Harris and Webb 1987).

Secure unit staff are 'in' secure accommodation too, and share the isolation, marginalisation and stigmatisation experienced by some of the children. Unless the careers of residential staff are taken more seriously, unless they are helped to develop professionally and rewarded for doing so, the abuses surfacing throughout residential care will almost certainly continue. Too many secure units constitute a shoestring facility, their size falling below that 'critical mass' necessary for reasonable facilities and companionship to be available. Units which provide a first-class service frequently do so by the willingness of exceptional individuals to accept low salaries, shift work, instability stemming from high staff turnover, and low status within their own agencies (for a further discussion of these points, see Utting 1991), and this is no basis for a facility such as secure accommodation. Although secure accommodation must perhaps remain ambiguous, it is possible for those involved with it to be helped to transcend this ambiguity. The alternative is to sink in a sea of confusion, perplexed at the meaning of the behaviours encountered, making mistakes and taking simplistic, punitive and sometimes illegal solutions.

5 Secure children?

> [F]ictional narratives and factual ones share the same episodic structure . . . we assimilate the written literature we read to the structure we use in our own oral narratives, the stories we tell about events that actually have happened to us. Of course, as we develop, this structure of narrative is undoubtedly affected by the stories we read or have read to us. In fact, this structure of personal narrative is probably formed by the stories to which we are exposed.
>
> (Peterson and McCabe 1983: 208)

> [A]fter writing three books to demonstrate that he was innocent of murder, and despite the endorsement of so influential a public figure as William F. Buckley, Jr., Edgar Smith finally admitted his guilt after all. With this as precedent one might be wary of any offender's 'story'.
>
> (Bennett 1981: 243–4)

The part of the research which focused on the children themselves was called the 'criteria study' because it examined the interpretation and application of the admission criteria laid down in legislation. It covered eleven authorities and was in two phases: the first, the *retrospective phase*, which we do not report here, comprised a content analysis of the files of all cases where secure accommodation had been used following the introduction of the legislation; the second, the *interview phase*, involved discussions with the forty children in secure accommodation when we visited and with the significant decision makers in their cases. Each phase sought to trace the decision-making process, to compare what happened in different authorities and different cases, and to set the official 'account' against the child's tale.

In this chapter the children and professionals we met in the second phase tell their stories. Some major themes re-emerge, but in the words of the participants themselves, sometimes consciously, sometimes, for such is the nature of narrative, shrouded in the dramatic irony of the unconscious disclosure. Whether they are social services managers, field or residential social workers, probation officers or the children themselves, our interviewees are all narrators, variably 'truthful' no doubt, and variably aware of complexity, but all telling their tales not as reliable or omniscient reporters, but as actors in the drama itself, each offering a unique inflexion, a perspective which, though never complete, constitutes a necessary part of a complex whole. Even those who 'lie' tell much to the alert narratee, for what is a lie but signally truthful representation of the world not as it is but as the 'liar' would wish it to be?

Hence, in part at least, our differences with Ariès (in his substitutive historiography) and Harding (in her notion of competing value perspectives). For it is not that if we clear away this patch of weeds or that thicket we shall somehow find pure and unsullied soil. The weeds, rather, are an inextricable part of the totality, only superficially obstacles to clarity, for in the world with which we are engaging, clarity itself is a chimera.

The logocentric notion that there is a 'core', 'heart' or 'key' is an important part of our cultural, conceptual and therefore linguistic worlds. It certainly affected our interviewees. For example, several children caused their social workers much anxiety because no one could, in the words of one, 'get to the bottom of him' or, in those of another, 'find out what made him do it'. The price to be paid by anxiety-provoking children was often to stay in secure accommodation for as long as it took for them to be 'fathomed'. In one case, we were told that this would be about three years and cost a quarter of a million pounds.

We must set aside such variables as 'theory' and 'professional judgement' in understanding how workers make their judgements precisely because it is not in the nature of such theory and judgement to lead inexorably to one answer. Professionals almost never referred to 'theory', and 'judgement' was, as we shall see, frequently controversial. Differences among professionals were seldom resolved by theoretical debate, but on the basis of the relative organisational power and status of the combatants, pragmatic and financial considerations and the attitudes (real or anticipated) of relevant others such as police, magistrates and press. Knowledge, and hence action, as one would expect in an area so dominated by paradigmatic conflict that contradictory arguments can be put with none of them open to authoritative repudiation, was a product of power relations within the organisation itself.

The muddles and contradictions which surfaced in a number of interviews are not necessarily indicative of intellectual flaccidity; they may equally represent a less than wholly conscious acknowledgement of the complexity of managing the conflict between oppositional goods. Here is a probation officer reflecting on whether it is his job to be concerned with 'protecting the public' in the case of David Harding, whom we shall encounter later, a boy who has committed three indecent assaults on little girls. Training will have taught him that protecting the public is the court's job and that his main responsibility is to the offender. In the messy world of practice, however, things are not so simple, and we encounter once again secure accommodation as an ineffable 'something', a *deus ex machina* necessary to resolve the practice dilemma:

Q I notice you made a comment about protecting the public in your report. Did you see that as one of your functions in writing it?

A No, because I think I also said in the same sentence that David needed help, he needed something. (*Pauses*) I don't know, I heard that the little girl who was assaulted had had some behaviour problems herself since the incident which was assumed by the doctor to be a result of the incident, and as far as I was in a position to make any decision I wouldn't have felt happy with him being out.

It is not that the probation officer is too stupid to understand, but that he is reflecting the complexity of an ambiguous situation. That he has failed to transcend this ambiguity is obviously regrettable, but in this failure he most clearly demonstrates the nature of the problem with which he (as professional), David (as boy in secure unit) and we (as commentators on the drama) have to engage.

CHILDREN'S STORIES

Three boys: Michael, David and Richard[1]

In Chapter 3 we explored some of the ways in which narrative is used, some of the simple stories which, though instantly recognisable, become more complex under scrutiny, characterised more by the moral dilemmas of the classics than by the formulaic attributes of trash. The cases we have chosen are not selected as representative or typical of the youngsters in secure accommodation: indeed, such was the diversity of the children that it would be hard to find such cases. We have selected instead children on whom we have sound data and whose cases are most obviously relevant to our themes. Michael is a psychologically damaged boy whose 'care career' has probably exacerbated his difficulties and has certainly provoked intense conflict within the agency; David has committed three indecent assaults and, though no one quite knows what to do with him, he has provoked few disagreements; Richard is on remand, awaiting Crown Court trial on a very serious charge to which he intends pleading Not Guilty. Different cases, different problems, recounted according to different scripts, but all proffering different arguments for the same conclusion: the boy must stay in secure accommodation.

Case A: Michael Johnson

Michael Johnson is 16, a boy with long-term contact with the welfare authorities. His history of truancy dates back to the age of 9, he was received into care at age 10 and made subject to a full care order at 13. This led to a succession of short-term placements, to many of which he reacted by physical and sexual violence, repeated absconding and, most significantly, criminal damage (attempting to burn down a living unit in his community home). Unsurprisingly, though until recently he had only a trivial criminal record, this act culminated in a secure placement. Following a short stay in a 'holding' establishment, the Mitchell Unit, he was placed in Larch Hill, a long-term regional secure facility where he was expecting to stay for over a year. Attempts were, however, being made to find him a more therapeutic alternative, and he was moved back into an open facility, Meadowhill, where he did not help himself by absconding through a lavatory window while waiting for a court hearing. When recaptured the following day he was returned to Larch Hill Regional Secure Unit on a renewed authorisation.

We spoke to Michael in Larch Hill, to the head of the Mitchell Unit, the Principal Officer and Assistant Director of Social Services, who had both been key decision makers, and a former, very significant, social worker. Interviews were taped and these accounts are taken from the transcripts. Where prompting was needed or answers edited, the customary dots have sometimes been omitted; in the case of the social worker's slightly disjointed account a number of different answers have been grouped together for ease of reading. Otherwise narratives are verbatim and, we hope, true to the sense in which they were recounted to us.

Michael described his care history, which began when he was living in Robsonville (150 miles away). His placement, by Robsonville Council, in Greenfields Home, Swanshire, triggered a family move to the county. He described his moves thus, but with a complexity only half grasped by the interviewer – for who was it but Michael whose behaviour triggered these increasingly frantic responses from the authorities? The power of the powerless should not be under-estimated, even though it may be used in a manner destructive to self and others:

> Then they sent me to Greenfields. I liked that and then my mum and that moved down and I used to go back to Robsonville for the holidays and then I got fed up with that and then they sent me home

for the holidays and after about two weeks I got fed up with that and they sent me to foster parents for holidays and then after about six months I didn't like that and ran away from them and then they sent me to Meadowhill after that. I stayed at Meadowhill and Sunnybank for the holidays and that, and then Meadowhill I went to all the time, then Sunnybank, then Mitchell, then they sent me here and then this place sent me back to – what was it – Meadowhill and then Meadowhill sent me to Mitchell and Mitchell sent me back here.

Q You make yourself sound like a sack of potatoes the way you talk! 'They' just did all these things to you and you got carried around. What do you think about that?

A I didn't mind some of it but I didn't like some of it at all.

Michael's capacity to perplex the authorities was considerable: the Head of Mitchell Secure Unit told us:

> Michael is a very disturbed boy, a very lonely boy, very insular, can't make many relationships at all, some odd characteristics in his behaviour, I mean there was the fire episode; also at one of his previous homes there had been inappropriate sexual approaches really, which might have been down to ignorance, and also damage to animals – he was seen as really potentially quite a dangerous boy, quite a difficult boy. He found it difficult to talk about any problems. Sometimes he would not just stay in bed but curl up into a ball under a duvet in a foetal position and stay there for a very long time. He was a worrying boy, very very withdrawn and had very little in the world in the way of links. I had to stop him assaulting mother once – on many occasions he would simply refuse to see her. He also used to foul round the room on occasions and sometimes outside the window. We gave him a room with a toilet which solved it sometimes but not really. It was deeper than a medical problem, he was a very worrying boy. I don't think he'll ever really adjust. His future is very bleak. There isn't a pattern of fire raising in the sense that he hasn't done it before. There's just the one major fire: he attempted to burn a living unit down and there could have been people inside – in fact he did it during the half term when it was empty – so there isn't a pattern but once done there's always a fear he could return to it.

Michael, like other children in this section 'worries' the professionals who, determined to find the mythical 'key' to his problems, become anxious at their failure to do so and make renewed efforts while, naturally, retaining him in security. 'Security' in this sense takes on yet a further layer of ambiguity: it not only provides security from and for the children, but for staff too, and the Head's worry about the lack of a 'pattern' of fire raising in Michael's behaviour seems a part of this. Michael, having no 'pattern' of fire raising, cannot reasonably be predicted as likely to repeat the act. Nevertheless, the possibility that he might do so causes the decision makers both *political* and *psychological* worries. There is, however, a pattern of a different kind in Michael's behaviour which involves running away, hiding, acting irrationally and unpredictably. With David Harding, as we shall see, the worry is a specific one about a 'pattern' of indecent assaults, and the emphasis is accordingly on providing specialist treatment. With Michael, however, the problem is that 'the pattern' constitutes no pattern at all, but disparate, unpredictable and intellectually 'unreachable' forms of behaviour, vulnerable, however, to *post hoc* reinterpretation by press, public and politicians should a risk be taken and something go badly wrong.

The professionals normally attributed their failure to find the 'key' to a lack of specialist knowledge. A characteristic response to existential doubt was to refer the case to a psychiatrist on whose word they would then hang. This response, however, should not be read as signifying unqualified approbation, for medical staff embody not only socially sanctioned 'expertise' but also a rival and potentially threatening explanatory discourse. This discourse may, of course, be deemed empirically insufficient: in the case of Michael, for example, his condition is '*deeper* than a medical problem'.

More significantly, however, some social professionals expressed profound ambivalence about the application of medical science to youngsters' problems, regarding with suspicion something they called 'the medical model'. Several times 'the medical model' appeared as an explanatory framework initially to be rejected, but returned to *in extremis*. The following interchange illustrates the view that too close an enmeshment in the psychiatric wing of the carceral system, for all the superior expertise which it makes available, creates the very problems which the secure units are designed to avoid. However convenient the existence of a socially sanctioned form of superior expertise to which the most mysterious and worrying cases can be entrusted may be, that expertise appears simultaneously helpful and unhelpful:

> He would have been happier here, but the problem was we didn't feel we could get to the very base root of his problems. It could be that nowhere will. The YTC might, but he needed such specialised help he probably needed sort of specialist therapy in certain areas, possibly in a psychiatric setting. We were struggling as we do with all the children, to keep him within social services. Because once they go to the health service some of them won't come out again, so you're struggling to keep them classed as normal, and I do see that as something we struggle to do when we can.

Q Is that part of the purpose of having secure units in social services? To keep boys from the health and penal services?

A Yes.

Q So you see yourself as having a defensive strategy?

A Yes. I mean there's a danger in labelling. Some of these children could easily go into a psychiatric unit and be labelled – label themselves – as that for a very long time, so we do, because of the secure unit, sometimes accept children who might be better off with full psychiatric attention, but we try and keep them out of that and work on an individual, almost common-sense behaviour modification type programme with no drugs to see if it will work.

Anxieties of a different kind emerged when we interviewed Swanshire's Principal Officer. The researcher began, conversationally:

Q I'm going to see Michael in Larch Hill tomorrow.

A I hope he doesn't hit you. He had a go at the last person from Swanshire who went up to see him. He sees Swanshire Social Services as very responsible for his being there.

The Principal Officer had in fact been one of a minority of people in favour of placing Michael in an open therapeutic unit, Yule Lodge; but placement decisions were taken by the Assistant Director who, in consultation with other professionals and the Director, had overruled him, apparently for an amalgam of reasons, none of them theoretical:

> He had a pretty long history of disturbance going back a long way. There was very worrying behaviour at Meadowhill especially *vis-à-vis* women staff. He went then to Sunnybank and didn't settle there, then he came to the Mitchell and the Mitchell staff were extremely worried about the actual and latent violence in the lad. The conclusion was he needed continued secure accommodation, either YTC or Larch Hill Secure Unit in that order. The social worker didn't know him too well as he'd only just been allocated the case: I think he'd seen him twice or something like that.

Q You also pursued a therapeutic option at Yule Lodge?

A That was very much the social worker's thought, and we did discuss it very much later on when Michael had already gone to Larch Hill and I think the magistrates were indicating that they would not make another secure order. The administration got a bit awry because I think the Mitchell had proceeded direct to explore YTC admission with DHSS. Next thing was that I had the Director of the Youth Treatment Centre on the phone asking me to give the local authority's commitment to a placement there. So I felt rather miffed actually, because I hadn't had the time to consider, to weigh up, to come to a view and I don't like being pressured and they wanted to remove the boy within a very short time – 8 days. This was very unusual. I enquired whether the Mitchell had placed in that particular YTC before, and how were they progressing? So there were a lot of things I tried to home in on, and finally decided that Larch Hill could offer a good programme for this lad, was nearer to hand to enable the parents and social worker to maintain contact, and finally plumped for Larch Hill.

Q Was that on therapeutic grounds as well as the other factors?

A I was reasonably satisfied that Larch Hill could develop a good programme for the lad.

Q Is part of the function just a holding thing really, to keep him out of harm's way?

A I hadn't thought of Larch Hill just holding him out of harm's way.

Q Did finance come into it?

A That was a consideration: you've got to take that into account, but it mustn't be the primary thing.

A very different view came from the boy's former social worker, Mr Davison, for whom Michael's case caused serious conflict with the department. Of all the professionals we met, he alone had decided not only that Michael's problems *were* comprehensible and *could* be managed, but that he was the person to do it. Unlike the other professionals, who all portrayed Michael as a brooding and mysterious personage with uncontrollable rages and villainous propensities, the story he told was, precisely, that of the angel with a dirty face, whose innate goodness was concealed both by mischance and by others' insensitivity. The story begins with the assessment which led to Michael's admission to the Mitchell Unit:

> He was assessed on the same site where he caused all the damage and I was a bit at loggerheads with the objectivity of the assessment with the two being very incestuous – a lot of staff partnerships and married couples between the two units. I ended up being very antagonistic actually, it felt like me and Michael against the wealth of residential provision and getting absolutely nowhere. I felt he was inappropriately placed in the open unit in the first place. He absconded three times in his four week stay there and on the fourth time he'd done all the damage. It seemed like he was saying something and no one was listening. My first feeling was 'Whoah! how can we stop this grinding machinery?'
>
> The psychiatrist had said that he couldn't guarantee he wouldn't do it again – i.e. go berserk and set fire to something. The fire wasn't – he was never charged with arson. It was the tail end of something. Basically he

ended up breaking into the office to get some money to go back to see his friends, and I think it was the confiscated cigarettes and matches drawer and confronted with this he thought he'd – erm, you know – everything else. He'd flooded the top floor and there were bedrooms and things. Sorry, I'm jumping about, there's no cohesion but his criminal record up to that point was a couple of Mars bars from Woolworth's: it was a comedy of errors really. If you take out the criminal damage there really wasn't a criminal – I mean a confused lad: no one was saying – I agree he was a problem, but the way of dealing with it was where we all found ourselves at opposite ends of the scale. A few shopliftings, he'd wrecked his own bedroom.

[There were instances of sexual assault against other children:]

I think again this whole Oedipal complex needed looking at. The unit he was placed in was a very macho unit; the chap running it, smashing chap – his hobby is a comedy strong man act and if you can find a telephone directory that hasn't been ripped or something .... The whole atmosphere was very macho and poor Michael presented as very feminine. A lot of his mannerisms were very camp, but he just did get on with girls very much easier. I think we make an adult psychopath, that's what I felt the way we dealt with him. I'm thoroughly depressed about the whole thing.

[Michael was made subject to a secure authorisation and went to the Mitchell, while the discussions we have seen took place as to his long-term future:]

Then came the fateful day when the Mitchell had heard that a bed was available at the Youth Treatment Centre on that day. This left the head of the Mitchell in the position of saying to the Assistant Director that he could go. He, I think, was a bit dubious about the reputation of the YTC at that time and said basically 'no' – he could go to Larch Hill. The first thing I knew was the following day when I heard Michael was in transit to Larch Hill. I'd never mentioned the place to him, it wasn't anywhere we'd discussed in our meetings.

I found him to be quite a bright lad but incredibly stubborn. He just said at our first meeting 'you've got to get me out of here', and that's quite a strong plea and from that point on I did try.

[The stay at Larch Hill was difficult, and other facilities continued to be considered; the social worker had his own views as to what should happen:]

He needed an assessment at somewhere like the Tavistock Clinic, somewhere you could believe in, where somebody had really sussed him out, because he was a difficult lad and there were a lot of very fine qualities about Michael which were always so readily overlooked because of his bizarre behaviour.

[He was then turned down for various therapeutic settings through lack of motivation. This suited him, because all he really wanted was a flat of his own, and he began to develop the idea that rejections from various homes would help him get one:]

Then came the fatal day when he made his threats at Meadowhill and Meadowhill took him back to court again. I wasn't about but he was taken to court and basically told to run while he was waiting at court because they couldn't fit him in in the morning, they'd gone for lunch, came back after lunch to say that Michael had run. Michael's side of that was that they'd had it – you know, the staff at Meadowhill had said, 'Well, if you fancy running we're not going to chase you'. That was very dubious practice; anyway what two staff are doing letting one little lad disappear over lunch when they've got him in custody to appear in court in the afternoon I don't know. Michael was arrested near a friend's house that evening and went back to court on the following day. And of course, you know – 'absconding, nobody can hold on to this lad' – there was no question but another 21A. Back to Larch Hill.

He knew he was going to jip and the more he fights it the more they'll get him taped as a psychopath or a madman. He'd already done some things like throw some tools in the workshop, he threw some tools about the place, injured another lad quite badly I think, and his parents were going to sue Michael. I know I could be accused of over-identifying perhaps, of being too emotional, but it felt the whole system, the whole bureaucratic machinery had been put into motion and there was no way you could get a spanner in there to stop any of the wheels grinding him into a pulp. I tried everything. I had the Director in court once, saying, 'Look, I can't go along with this', but obviously her authority reigned supreme in that situation. All she'd say was 'I've discussed this with colleagues and we feel this is the best place for him'. That was the blanket response.

I didn't have a downer on secure accommodation, in fact it's my background. They have their uses and I just felt it wasn't that I had any bone to pick with the secure centres or anything. And when those amounts of financial resources are being talked about, my mind was going crazy, I mean could I be given a year off, you know, £8,000 a year doesn't go anywhere, and I'll just have this one client – I was desperate to try anything because you could just see that in that situation he was just one of those lads who would self-destruct because of this stubborn streak, he will push that structure to its limits. And he knew all the tricks: you know if you poured a cup of boiling hot tea over someone it was

> looked on much more seriously than if you threw a glass of water over someone or tipped the table over.

Superficially this is a simple and moving tale. The social worker is Mr Brownlow, thwarted in his attempts to help Oliver. It is not, however, easily encapsulated, for Mr Davison can sustain it only by under-playing, indeed dismissing, the concerns of more senior staff about Michael's dangerousness, and the dangerousness is, after all, a necessary part of this complex tale. The social worker, however, not only locates the causes of Michael's problems firmly in external factors – family relationships, care history – but also makes a rescue bid: he will take the boy over and save the authority money in the process, becoming as it were the *deus ex machina* of a thousand novels and dramas. Note the dramatic terminology of the comedy of errors, fateful and fatal days, the comic character who tears up telephone directories, the hint of conspiracy, even skulduggery, while Michael struggles to maintain his dignity, even perhaps his sanity, against the 'grinding machinery' moving inexorably to destroy him.

Behind it all, however, lies a particular and contradictory image of Michael. He is indeed fighting the system, but he is close also to severe mental illness. He should go to 'somewhere like the Tavistock Clinic' (the significant 'somewhere' emerging once more) or he may become a psychopath. And the destructive behaviour is all the time minimised: throwing tools in a workshop, even throwing boiling tea instead of a glass of cold water over someone are reported not as dangerous assaults but merely in terms of their supposed 'meaning' for Michael and their likely consequences for him; hence the one leads to possible court action while the other is a piece of effective manipulation.

Michael's own explanation of his most serious act, fire raising, was telic: it was an opportunistic but unsuccessful attempt to manipulate the system as though he too, like Mr Davison, saw himself as 'against the world'. He was already predisposed to hostility, perceiving himself a victim of injustice: clearly, even open community homes are characterised by the inaccuracies and injustices of a closed system:

> I went into the office at Meadowhill and looked at my file, and all things what I was supposed to have done, the bad things mainly, and all the reasons why I was placed with them and it was all rubbish and I could have writ it better myself and people had writ it that I didn't even know and had never even seen – he was writing reports on me and I didn't know nothing about them, he didn't know nothing about me and he was writing them on me as well. I talked to staff about it but they says oh, you couldn't have got in there because it was locked.

Q So they thought you were lying?

A Yeah.

Q But you weren't?

A (*Laughs*) No! And they knew I weren't because I could see things and they went and checked to see if they were right. They knew I wasn't but they didn't admit it.

In his *naïveté* Michael believed that to set fire to the unit would speed his discharge:

I hated Sunnybank. You never used to do anything, just sit around. The staff were horrible, not nice to anybody.

Q So you burnt it down. I can't quite work that out Michael – it's a funny thing to do to get bored and burn the place down.

A I didn't go there intending to do it I went there planning to abscond and get some money, so I just went there and smashed the window and I was trying to knock this thing out and I found some matches, and I smashed loads of windows to start off with. Then I thought I'll be able to get into the Mitchell and I'll only have to stay there a few months and get home, so I thought that's better than staying here for a year or something, so I did that, and then I see some matches so I just set fire to it.

His knowledge of the system, however, though characterised by a bewildering grasp of detail, is partial. Michael himself seems to know that he lacks the calculative ability ultimately to win. His life is measured out not in coffee spoons but in three-month sequences, sequences which have a profound impact on his own time-scales:

Q What are they going to do with you now?

A Dunno. I've been here for about nine months this time and I've had three case conferences and the first one they said you're allowed out, and then I absconded and they said at the second you'll have to wait three months again and I committed an offence that time and you have to wait three months if you commit an offence and if you don't it's only two months, and then I absconded again and committed another offence and had to wait three months, and I was allowed out again and about a month later I absconded and I didn't commit any offences so I've got to wait about another month now. If you're making progress you're supposed to be going out all the time and going on home leaves and that and I don't do none of that, I just stick about a couple of times and then abscond. You have to go out with a member of staff first of all, you know, and then they'll let you out on your own if you're lucky.

Q Why do you run away if you know that if you don't run away they'll let you out?
A 'Cos three months seems a long time.

Michael's explanation of his plight is, like that of his social worker – and, did he know it, the Dartington researchers too (Millham *et al.* 1978) – situational, related to the failings of the care system rather than to personal pathology. He sees himself as a victim of circumstance; that he is a young criminal he does not deny; that he would have been otherwise had he not been dealt with as he was is his contention. This account offers, of course, a narrative resolution of the moral dilemma we discussed in Chapter 3, of what is to be done with the youngster who, though deprived and sad, is none the less recalcitrant. Michael's answer is to do less, his dictum *primum non nocere*, avoid iatrogenesis, but it is an answer which reflects his interests, not his needs. It does, however, address his 'rights' in so far as he perceives them to have been abrogated by the coercion to which he has been and still is subject: his bad acts are only bad acts in a context which oppresses and is destroying him; his political position is close to being revolutionary:

Q Are you saying that if you hadn't been nicked for stealing the sweets, and you hadn't gone into care, you wouldn't have any problems?
A No, I would have problems but not as many. I probably wouldn't be in a secure unit. It's when you go into children's homes, it's not the same as home because in the family bit you don't have anybody nicking stuff and that, but in the children's homes nearly everybody's doing it and you learn new things. You get worse in here as well: people come in here for different things; there's always something to learn about and then you know them so you probably go and try it out yourself. (*Laughs*)
Q But you're not in the secure unit for that but for setting fire to Sunnybank. You wouldn't have done that if you hadn't been in there?
A I wouldn't have had any reason to do it if I hadn't been in there.
Q So partly you're here because care has made you worse?
A Yeah.

Yet even this is not simple, for remember how he was physically restrained from attacking his mother and how he refused to see her. And further, in an ironic twist, when we asked him if he wanted to leave he said not yet: he was taking school examinations in the summer and was in the middle of his course work. If successful he hoped to go to a further education college and train to be a teacher. The compulsion to which he was subject seemed a necessary precondition for Michael to have any chance of success. Ambiguity and complexity indeed.

Case B: David Harding

David Harding is a 15-year-old boy with no previous care history, though he has been subject to probation supervision for the first of three indecent assaults on young girls. The assaults occurred in a relatively short space of time and were of escalating seriousness, the attacks becoming graver and the victims younger. He was made subject to a secure accommodation authorisation for the third of these offences, and the problem now is what to do with him. Like Michael, David has the unfortunate habit of alarming the authorities who, because they do not 'understand' him, do not trust him. The scope for demonstrating trustworthiness in a secure unit is, however, limited, and this dilemma is especially highlighted in this case.

Unlike Michael, David has no Brownlow to support him. Unlike Michael too he is an unattractive boy and his ugliness seems, unsurprisingly, to be held against him: villains are frequently ugly and frequently threatening. David exerts the power of the powerless over his professionals, but, as with Michael, that power is redirected by its recipients and used to justify further control over him. His unit manager describes him thus:

> He's a strange looking boy, he's got very staring eyes, he is balding at barely 15, losing quite a lot of his hair – both tendrils are well back, about 3–4 inches. He came in with a beard and a moustache – he looks about 23; he's got staring eyes which at first made us quite uneasy, though they don't now. You tend to think that if it was half light and you found this lad standing over you you would be petrified: he's a very strange looking boy, a very odd looking boy, very strange.

He makes others nervous too, sometimes just at the level of a 'feeling' defying precise explanation. His probation officer said:

> It worried me, it was a worrying case. David worried me because I always found him very cold, a very cold lad. I mean he cooperated a hundred per cent, he was one of the most brilliant reporters I've ever had on a supervision order, he never failed to keep an appointment and he was always prompt, he was always *there* basically, but I just felt him rather cold, I can't think of a better word to describe it really.
>
> Q Was that a hunch you had, or was it based on any behaviour he showed?
>
> A I guess he didn't really show a lot if any remorse for what he'd done. I think I put in one set of notes that I'd really like to get through to

> what he thinks, what he's actually thinking, instead of giving me the answers that he thinks I want to hear to the questions I posed. I felt that very strongly.

Again here we encounter this urge to 'get through', which all the professionals we spoke to shared, and in a manner inextricably linked to their perceptions of risk. The quest is there for sufficient understanding to render David harmless, but the quest is a long-term one and it is not entirely clear how, even if it were completed, success would be recognised and acknowledged. The characteristic result of ever-deepening social enquiry is not the discovery of successful solutions but the uncovering of more problems. This has obvious consequences for David's discharge. These comments from the head of unit demonstrate first that the staff are floundering, secondly that as a result they are relying unquestioningly on the psychiatrist's superior expertise to determine whether David should stay or go, and thirdly that the technical problem of demonstrating whether David is dangerous or not while he is in secure accommodation is considerable:

> This is a worrying case. The great problem is trying to evaluate his level of dangerousness in a secure provision where he can't repeat the offence. After the second offence he had a considerable amount of therapy and guidance on the sexual matters from a specialist, and it was hoped that this would cure things, but it didn't – it doesn't seem to have made a great deal of difference.
>
> David is a very dull, withdrawn sort of boy, can't make relationships at all, tries very hard, is permanently at the bottom of the pecking order, as it were, in here, and there are some quite inadequate children in here anyway. We've taken him through a whole battery of medical tests via the psychiatrist hoping to find something which would indicate why he was behaving in this way. But they're all proving normal, and at the moment we're worrying around how much of a risk he is and whether he ought to go secure.
>
> We're really not sure which way to go, but the psychiatrist is recommending extreme caution, so really we haven't got beyond the first hurdle of whether he's going open, with intensive staff support, or do we need the additional backup of a secure unit to make sure he doesn't slip away from this? On balance the specialist thinks that he needs secure.

Q Does this uncertainty go back to the evidential problem of how you assess dangerousness in a secure unit?

A Yes.

Q And how do you? By depending on the specialist's opinion?

A The specialist's opinion, the psychiatrist's opinion.
Q And do you have any worries about the status of that, the competence of that?
A No, we're lucky.

David is so well behaved, so conformist, that everyone believes him to be 'putting on an act'. Of course we all 'put on acts' all the time, selecting the modes of self-presentation which seem appropriate or strategic, but David lacks the subtlety to do it successfully. A partial recognition of this point on the part of the professionals leads to a theory of David's delinquency which owes less to psychopathology than to social skills. So dominant is the former mode of explanation, however, that even this new theory is translated into the idea that David needs an unusual and highly specialised form of sex therapy:

> The trouble [*sic*] with David is he's no management problem at all; he's a quiet withdrawn boy who can't express his feelings. There are girls here he tries to make relationships with, but he doesn't get very far because there are more personable lads who come in and lift them off him. He certainly is not a physical boy in terms of aggression; in fact he would back away if his girlfriend were taken off him. So he can't make relationships: what does he do? He goes out and finds younger girls and he makes approaches to them, clumsy approaches which then become physical assaults.

Q He sounds as though he needs a girlfriend of his own!
A Yes, or perhaps some sexual therapy – with a woman, you know, a woman who is available, and available in physical terms.

Clearly this point has been much discussed by the professionals. When the 'girlfriend' point was put to his field social worker the same suggestion emerged, this time couched in terms of social learning:

Q What would you say to the rather flippant suggestion that what he really needs is a girlfriend of his own?
A (*Laughs awkwardly*) You see I don't think that's flippant because it's something that I have suggested. I didn't think of it in terms of a girlfriend because I don't think a girlfriend is going to be experienced enough to deal with his problems. (*Laughs*) I don't know who's going to hear this tape or what they're going to think of what I'm going to say, but what I felt was that if there was some sexual therapist who could teach him how to deal with a sexual relationship in a more usual form, combined with feeling and caring – I mean I don't know how feasible that is – he is more likely at a later date to have a sexual relationship combined with feelings and love. The

> great fear I have is that if he succeeds in having sex with somebody in a rape situation the buzz he's going to get out of that is going to be almost impossible to change. If he can get a buzz out of a sexual therapist he is more likely to steer away from having to rape somebody to get the buzz I think he's after.

Everyone not so much 'puts on' an act as plays a part all the time, with varying degrees of sophistication and success; we present ourselves in certain ways, engage in impression management or information control (Goffman 1963, 1968), and like the rest of us Michael and David inevitably engaged in these activities, though they received startlingly different responses. David provokes more uniform responses than Michael, precisely because he is such a stereotypically recognisable character, the schoolboy creep, a physically unpleasant and scapegoated child who curries favour but then sneaks to others, a boy with minor but noticeable physical defects such as bad breath, a tendency to perspire and acne, and with nervous habits such as picking spots, biting nails and scratching. The motif is most immediately from schoolboy fiction of the nineteenth and twentieth centuries, but the character has a long and predominantly comic literary pedigree, the most celebrated instance being Fielding's Master Blifil in *The History of Tom Jones*. The only truly sympathetic response to David was from his probation officer in responding to the suggestion that he might, instead of being committed to a secure unit, have gone to detention centre. His response was strong, unequivocal and protective:

> Detention centre would have been absolutely devastating for David. It wouldn't have equipped him with social skills, he would have been picked upon, bullied, and as soon as the boys found out what he was in there for – and I'm sure a few obliging prison officers would have told them – I think he'd have been beaten up and received all the usual cruelties that kids like that do receive. I can just imagine David lying in a ball in the corner in a dreadful state.

The authorities, meanwhile, were embarking with vigour on their quest for the perfect therapeutic regime. Apparently the unit where David was being held was not offering therapy of an appropriate kind, but the decision had still to be taken as to whether David should, in the words of the manager, 'go secure or go open'. This decision was dependent first on the opinion of the psychiatrist, who had still to make up his mind, and secondly on the availability of resources. If the ideal therapeutic environment was secure David would 'go secure', if not, he would 'go open'. The question of 'secure or open' was hence subordinated to the exigency of finding the right therapy. David's social worker, however, who described to us a bewildering array of institutions he was visiting to assess the suitability of their various therapeutic regimes for David, appeared decidedly confused. By chance, on the day of our visit the social worker had just secured a six-month renewal of David's secure authorisation. We asked him why:

> Because we're still in the process of assessing his needs. I think to some extent we've assessed where David is at but I don't think we've fully assessed the resources that are going to be available for him. So I suppose really what we presented to the court this morning was a combination of both those needs, mainly through looking on the side of resources as opposed to knowing what David needs. I suppose it's a matter of finding the right place for him. The reports we've had so far suggest that sex counselling is the sort of area his needs are going to be in.
>
> What we did this morning was we explained to the court that part of the treatment is an ongoing assessment, part of that is finding out exactly what we can offer David in terms of where his needs can be met. The psychiatric report made it very clear that this was a dangerous boy who is more than likely to reoffend. He seems to be an opportunist in as much as there is no real concern about him running away from the unit and committing an offence but if he's in a situation in which he can commit an offence he will do that.

David had no criminal history prior to his commission of the three sexual offences in adolescence. These, however, combined with his physiognomy to suggest to the professionals that his pathology was amenable only to specialised therapeutic modes, not to the 'common-sense behaviourism' of the secure unit. Nevertheless, his response to authority was to conform entirely, to manifest no disturbance (other than of a social kind): on probation he was a 'brilliant reporter', and in secure accommodation, at one, but only one, level, a model resident. The problem was acknowledged:

> He's made no move here against anybody at all. He goes out on mobility with staff and sticks so closely to them that he trips them up, literally. I worry a bit when he's out but really there's no need and it's a very artificial situation. The real way to test him, which wouldn't be responsible, would be to put him back in his home for the weekend or a week and give him an awful lot of freedom – and you'd then find out, perhaps, at someone else's expense. And perhaps you'd need longer. He was put here because someone decided that wasn't right. Most sexual offences are decided by the courts, which takes the onus off us. But this offence is difficult to get hold of, what its content was, what his intentions were – would he have stopped? It's a nebulous offence to pin down.

So what does he have to do to get out? We put this question to all the decision makers, and all, not surprisingly, found it hard to answer. The unit manager:

> In the end someone will have to take the decision – this boy's potentially dangerous therefore we cannot go open, and I think that decision will be taken by myself in consultation with the psychiatrist and people from County Hall, looking at all the evidence. We have to be guided by the psychiatrist. Nothing we've seen here suggests he is a dangerous boy, but it's a very artificial way of living.
>
> Q So what would he have to do to get out?
>
> A (*10-second pause*) That's a good question. I think he'd need to be able to talk about his problems, which he's not very skilled at doing because he is a dull boy with an IQ about 70–75. I think he'd need to convince the sexual therapists who'd worked with him, the specialists, that he had absorbed their help, the counselling they're offering him, which he hadn't earlier. And maturity? – he's quite a mature boy in some respects anyway. It's a good question. I think really reassure people over a longer term, perhaps just the passage of time – which doesn't give him a lot to work at, does it?

The Assistant Director:

> Q One of the issues is 'how does he get out?'
>
> A It is difficult. My understanding is he's physically well developed but has a mental age well below his chronological age. So the basic worry is that he's not able to exercise any degree of control over his behaviour, and how do you build on what he's got is the basic point.

And the social worker:

> Q What's he got to do to get out?
>
> A (*Laughs*) That's a very fair question: do you want me to try to answer it? What he's got to do to come out is show us that what he's learned and how he presents make the people dealing with him feel he's not going to be a threat to young girls outside. That I think is going to be a fairly long-term process but it will include giving him rope but which doesn't include 'one day you're locked up the next you're not'. It'll involve actually working with him on his offending and his having to recognise that. Then alongside that expanding if you like or increasing his mobility.
>
> Q When do you guess that process might begin?
>
> A I don't think it can begin until there is a structured approach to

working with him and his behaviour. I don't think that's actually happening in the unit. I think they would agree with me. Obviously there is counselling but not what I would call confrontation going on to the extent that there would be in some sort of treatment centre.

Q Is he then being held partly because of the therapeutic deficiencies of the unit?

A I wouldn't see it as being a therapeutic unit. My understanding of their role is to make an assessment. It's inevitable that in the course of doing that there is going to be feedback to David, but I don't see that as a key part of their role.

If we cannot measure future intentions by present behaviour, especially in a supposedly opportunist offender such as David, it is difficult to make predictive decisions. What emerges is not a decision based on quantitative measurement, for such a calculation is theoretically and empirically impossible. Hence the issue becomes bureaucratic, based less on a calculation of the risk the boy presents than the risk to the agency of any particular course of action. The unit manager again:

> David is our problem. If after three cases like this he were placed open and some little girl was raped there would be an outcry: why was he allowed to do it again? If it was burglary or cars you might take the risk, but when you're talking about fires or sexual offences you have to be very careful.

Part of David's problem is, however, that precisely by *not* 'opening up' to his professional helpers he is mounting a challenge to the very basis of their supposed expertise. Talking cures cannot work unless the patient talks, and when a crypto-therapeutic relationship is resisted by silence or exaggerated conformity, the confidence of the workers begins to be undermined. *Their* script is that they are the benign helpers of sad or destructive youngsters. For the youngster's script to involve silent survival in an incomprehensible world is to draw the teeth of the theoretically powerful professionals by rendering them therapeutically powerless. It is, however, a characteristic consequence for the flexing of their muscles by the powerless to rebound on them, and in this case the child is to remain in security until he follows the correct script. We put this point to David's social worker, perhaps a little discourteously. It was answered in terms of the need for openness: ironically, one enters open accommodation through openness. Further, however, and in a further exemplification of one of our seven dilemmas, the boy may be so damaged that he actually wants to stay:

Q What if somebody said that he didn't say anything because he's not very bright or articulate, he doesn't understand abstractions about treatment and training and just wants to get out? One could say it's hard for him to answer that question in the way the professionals want him to. Has he actually got to learn the therapeutic ropes?

A I think what we've always tried to do in terms of his own limited understanding is explain to him what we're doing and why we're doing it. One of the important things is that they have to have some understanding of what the hell we're doing. He likes being in the unit: in fact, he is secure [*sic*] and happy there. That in itself isn't going to help him in the long term.

If the professionals, confused as to how to proceed and using the psychiatrist to legitimate holding a boy who lacks the practical power to 'earn' his discharge, are nevertheless caused serious anxiety, what does David himself make of it all? The interview began with a burst of loquacity and humour, but as this was not maintained it is likely to have been a well-prepared opening, involving a self-deprecating and pre-emptive reference to his physical appearance. David was asked about his first day in the unit:

> I'll tell you something. When I was talking to one of the staff as I had my dinner it just looked all weird to me as it's the first time I've been in care, and I was sitting in the dining room with one of the staff and talking to her and all the kids was staring at me – because they thought I was a social worker! And I'm only 15.

Beyond this his responses were mainly monosyllabic and punctuated by lengthy silences. This extract is the most painful part of the interview. David, possibly over-led by the interviewer, is describing his own lack of knowledge as to how he will behave in the future:

Q Do you remember the first hearing at all?
A No.
Q Had you ever heard of secure accommodation before?
A No.
Q Tell me now what you think it is.
A I think it's a place where people can help you. To make sure the person doesn't do it again.
Q So you see it as stopping you committing the offences again. Is that why you're here, do you think?
A Yes.
Q Why locked up?
A If you're locked up you can't go out and do it again.
Q Do you think that's fair?
A Yes.

Q So if they went to court and asked for a 6-month renewal what would you think about that?
A I don't know about that. I'm not sure. I wouldn't mind going home.
Q When do you think they'll let you out?
A Not for some time yet.
Q Why is that?
A The offences I suppose, in case I go and do it again.
Q Have you been interviewed by a lot of people in here, psychiatrists and people, who ask you whether you are going to do it again? And what do you tell them?
A I promise them I'll never do it again. I've said that to everybody.
Q But do you think you might do it again?
A (*Grunts*)
Q Is that right? You say to them you won't do it again to get out, but secretly you think you might do it again?
A Yes.
Q Are you worried about that?
A (*Sotto voce*) A bit, yeah.
Q But you can't talk to them about it?
A No.
Q Why not? (*17-second pause*) Because if you do – what? (*7-second pause*) They might not let you out? (*Apparently nods*) Yes, I can see that. That's a terrible situation to be in, isn't it? Does it wind you up sometimes or do you not bother?
A (*Immediately*) I don't bother.

Case C: Richard Miles

This is a strange case. He claims that he didn't commit the offence, he wasn't there at the time. This is being supported by a family alibi. He's been picked out on identity parade by the girl but the forensic evidence is negligible. The weapon has never been found and Richard is claiming a case of mistaken identity. So we've been mainly a remand facility in this case, partly an assessment unit too, but it's difficult to assess the boy because he's maintaining events which are alleged to have happened didn't happen at all. You don't quite know what you're assessing. Within the unit he's been himself, slightly cocky, unworried, which astonishes the staff, completely unworried, assured that in fact he'll be out by Christmas and have his Christmas dinner at home.

We were given the option of taking him as it was a very serious offence. If we'd declined to do so he would have gone to the remand centre. Having said that, that's what we're here for, to take children like this, and we can't back off from the difficult ones. The only thing would be if the other children were safe with him. He's not been a boy who worries staff, though he's a deep boy, there are undercurrents to him that we feel we haven't completely got to.

Q So you are in effect an extremely expensive holding facility?'

A Yes.

Q What do you think about that?

A (*Pause*) In this case (*pause*) I think it's reasonable in this case because although we haven't done a psychiatric investigation we have built up quite a picture of the boy through psychological testing, and the feeling is that even if he's found Not Guilty, which seems increasingly likely, that he might go into voluntary care, because the home situation has some difficulties. So what we found out in this case might be useful for voluntary care proceedings [*sic*].

We shall say less about Richard Miles because the issues raised by the case, though complex to unravel, are simpler to express. Richard's alleged offence was the attempted murder by multiple stabbing of a young woman. He denied the offence and was on remand in a secure unit rather than in a penal establishment.

Like the two youngsters already discussed, Richard caused much worry to his professionals, again for reasons they could not quite quantify. This surfaced in comic form in an encounter narrated by his social worker:

He used to work part time – weekends presumably – at a local butcher's shop.

Q (*Cheerfully*) Well, if he's found Guilty that would be quite appropriate!

A (*Laughs*) That's right! I found that out sat in the back of a Panda car going up to Eastville, making general conversation with Richard, and asked him what his interests were, and he said butchery! . . . Whether he said it for effect I don't know.

Like David, Richard refused to play a part in the therapeutic script. This refusal led to much probing into his background, and the more the professionals probed the more they found and the more justifications consequently emerged for holding Richard in a unit geared to individualised helping if not therapy. A senior manager was alert to the complexities of this, seeking nevertheless to establish, for reasons which were unclear, whether Richard's family believed in his innocence:

In a unit as small as ours there were very obvious problems in Richard's life to be addressed, and we wanted some permission from Richard's parents to address them rather than say, 'Oh, we can't do anything'. And in fact Richard's parents did say, 'Yes, by all means do what you can: we think there are problems as well', but having said that they were still maintaining his innocence. If this were my child and I were so convinced of his innocence I would be asking for bail. What I was really trying to do was test out whether the parents really believed in his innocence or not. It didn't ring true somewhere or other. But we said that we would look at our other children's facilities in other parts of the county. And having said that, Mr Williams the social worker went away and made enquiries about other facilities and they were all too scared to have him.

Q So it was 'Guilty until proved innocent'?

A Well that's very much so, yes. People are very afraid of Richard. It was rather tacky circumstances surrounding that case.

Richard's social worker touched on this and other themes, some of them already the familiar ones of the awkward relation between needs and rights, the practice of professional pathology hunting within the family, the notion that there is a core problem which it is the professional task to penetrate, and the notion that 'need' can be unrecognised by the needer and accessible only to specialist therapeutic expertise:

> It's awful unfair because it means we're prejudging the thing but I think we're all a bit worried about Richard and feel that there's a lot of work there to be done, but because he's not admitted the crime – and OK we can't know for certain whether he has – (*voice trails off*) – it's very difficult for the unit to work with him, because until it comes out in the open they can't, you know, get behind it. They *are* doing their best to help him there, and there's quite a few bits that have come out about the family and home life. I feel that household isn't particularly a happy one. Though on the surface everything's bright and wonderful, they won't actually let very much out. I mean if they are actually lying to provide an alibi for Richard I suppose they've got to keep things very tight so they don't let anything slip. But I think there's an awful lot going on in that family that we need to get to the bottom of to help Richard and possibly his brother – he does need treatment, he does need help. He's not accepting it but I think he *needs* it, and I feel personally that if anybody can give it to him it is in that sort of closed situation. I think your average children's home – and I've worked in residential care – wouldn't be able to give him the kind of support that he needs.

At the time of the research (though this has subsequently been changed) the period spent on remand was not deducted from any future custodial sentence, and Richard, though not a talkative boy, was well aware of the 'justice' dimension of this:

> I haven't got a clue why I'm here, even though I know the case I'm on. If I'm innocent I don't know why I'm in secure accommodation this far away from home.
>
> Q That's the unfair bit is it, being so far from home?
>
> A Yes. I'm innocent until I'm proven guilty, but they – unit and police – are saying I'm guilty until I'm proven innocent.
>
> Q So why do you think they are locking you up?
>
> A I know what they're on about. It's doing my head in.

Richard's case presents another dilemma: he cannot 'discuss his problems' because in so far as they relate to an offence which he denies, none exists. He is in secure accommodation only because it is deemed preferable to a prison or remand centre, but because he is being held by staff with a therapeutic orientation he is being subjected to a form of personal scrutiny he appears not to want, and is now even being discussed, in the event of an acquittal, as a possible candidate for voluntary care. The unit's *raison d'être* involves personalised counselling with acknowledged problems, but Richard either does not have or cannot discuss any such problems. And the financial burden of his containment falls on (as they then were) the rate-payers, whereas had he been held, as he could have been, in a remand centre, the cost would have been borne entirely by central government. Richard does on the face of it appear to have paid a considerable price for the fact that secure accommodation is not quite prison.

Two girls: Karen and Sarah

A number of girls featured in our study. Though numerically in a minority, girls are of interest precisely because the very ambiguity of secure accommodation which we have been discussing may take on a different inflexion in their case. We know from previous research that girls, though more likely to be kept out of the justice and care systems in the first place are, once inside the system, liable to be propelled more quickly than boys into tutelary disposals on grounds which reflect a generalised concern about their welfare needs and sexual conduct (Harris and Webb 1987: ch. 6; Harris 1992: ch. 5).

We asked about girls when we spoke to the social service managers in the first phase of the study. We sometimes gained the impression that we were touching on a delicate issue, and the predominant response was to claim that, while girls did indeed have different problems, they were, presumably in the interests of sex equality, dealt with in the 'same way' as boys. To deal with different problems in the same way is not, however, obviously rational, as is perhaps reflected in the defensiveness of this response:

> There are quite a number of girls admitted. Girls can be quite frightening and difficult to handle.
>
> Q Are there different criteria for girls?
>
> A The circumstances will be different. You're not talking about cases of a lot of burglaries, but 'out of control', 'moral danger', 'arson'. So the presenting problems – but we're certainly not going to say, 'Oh, girls need protecting more than boys'.

When we asked the girls about the issue we received a variety of responses. What follows, from a difficult but not heavily delinquent 15-year-old, was among the most interesting because it so precisely pinpointed a number of ambiguities which cause operational difficulty: treating people individually versus treating them identically; 'trusting' people who have in the past been untrustworthy versus acting on the basis of a realistic prediction of future behaviour; explicitly managing the material and biological differences between boys and girls versus acting in a way which cannot be said to involve gender bias:

> But say a boy went on the run, he wouldn't get into as much trouble as a girl would. This lad I used to go out with, he went on the run 32 times from the kids' home. I went on the run 3 or 4 times and I got sent away. That's wrong. They should be treated equally. A lad can get into more trouble than a girl can. They are worried about girls getting pregnant and going into prostitution, and things like that.
>
> Q Are they right to be worried?
>
> A In a way yes, in a way no. If they know the girl they shouldn't just jump to conclusions. They should think, because that could upset a girl, thinking she could do this, she could do that. They could drive her mental.

In this section we feature two girls whose victimisation is manifest but whose actions have compounded their personal tragedies. The relationship between tragic circumstance and destructive act, being a case study in the broader arguments about the nature of freedom, is not ultimately determinable, but, as we have seen, secure accommodation must, irrespective of such considerations, encompass all the otherwise uncontainable problems which children present. Neither of these girls fits into the simple literary motifs of Chapter 3, but each of them presents particular challenges to the child-care system.

Case D: Karen Jarvis

Karen is a 15-year-old girl who has been in the care system for a number of years following a series of disputes with her mother and a succession of her mother's cohabitees. This is her first experience of a secure unit. We spoke to the head of the unit where Karen was living, her social worker and Karen herself. The social worker gave us a detailed account of Karen's life; this extract is typical:

> The situation at home broke down. She had been missing from home on several occasions and her mother asked for voluntary care. She was placed at an observation and assessment unit and appeared to settle down for a time. Mother then herself disappeared. There was no way I could control Karen for a few weeks after that. She sent word then that she was coming to collect Karen. Now the relationship between Karen and her mother left a lot to be desired. Mother was not the type of person able to offer the affection and love which the girl was apparently craving. Consequently Karen was reported to me by her parents – her mother, natural father – staff at the school and others as being a promiscuous girl who gravitated to any lad who showed her the least crumb of affection. So she was a very promiscuous girl according to all reports that had been given to me.
>
> Mother sent word from her new house (100 miles away) to say 'I'm coming to take Karen back; I have re-established contact with my cohabitee and I want her to come with me'. Karen immediately panicked – 'There's no way I'm going'. At her age you have to have some respect for what the young person wants; you've got to give some consideration – you can't say 'You *are* going'. In a case like this I felt quite strongly that in view of what she was saying we had to consider what she was saying and, if necessary, take the case back before the courts, and go for an interim care order to stop Mum from removing her from care.
>
> So I went over, saw Karen, said 'Look, don't go'. She started to threaten she was going to abscond. I said 'Don't be silly. Stay here over the weekend, nothing will happen. We will take whatever steps are necessary to stop Mum from coming to take you to remove you from care. I contacted the mother and more or less told her the same, so the mother said 'All right, I shall not come until the Monday'. In the mean time Karen absconded. She was missing for quite a lengthy period of time, nearly a month on that occasion. She was picked up by the police, living with a girl in a nearby seaside resort. They had made a complaint that someone had gone into the flat and tampered with the electricity meter. She was living under an assumed name, had dyed her hair and had gone to some lengths to try to hide her identity. But unfortunately for her

> the police officer who visited the home knew her from school! Of course, he recognised her, but said later she was very convincing in her denial. He took her in.
>
> Incidentally, she always denied she had been sexually involved, but she had two packets of condoms and a packet of birth control pills. It's fair to assume she was sexually involved at that time. So then she admitted she had a boyfriend. She'd seen a number of different boys. Her memory's very short-lived. She was brought back on that occasion, said she wasn't staying and absconded within a relatively short period of time.

The situation was complicated in Karen's case because she claimed to have been absconding from an open unit (which she disliked) precisely in order to enter secure accommodation: a dilemma for the professionals which we have already noted. Karen told the researcher, in yet a further instance of the power of the powerless:

> I hated the place; I didn't want to stay.
>
> Q Had you anywhere you wanted to get to?
>
> A Yes, I wanted to get here. I loved this place even though I'd only been here one night. I just like it the way it is. I knew if I kept running away I'd get a secure order on me, because my social worker had said.

While she was away the staff feared she was surviving by prostitution and sought to use secure accommodation to protect her from this behaviour in a way that no open facility seemed able to. She too, in the arguments of the professionals, is a girl who, never having learned legally or morally acceptable modes of conduct, needs the artificial boundary of secure accommodation to make her learn without fleeing. More than this, however, secure accommodation for Karen is a retreat, an asylum, in which, by private contemplation and counselling, she can again 'place' herself, physically and morally, in a bewildering world:

> One girl, who she ran with on most occasions, said to staff that Karen had said to her that if she needed extra finance she was able to raise it. So you can read into that what you want.
>
> Q So there were serious questions about prostitution?
>
> A Very serious. I honestly felt I had to protect that girl.
>
> Q And you were using secure accommodation for her own protection more than anything else?
>
> A Yes, but she demanded it . . .
>
> Q Do you think that the restrictions on the use of secure accommodation are helpful or not helpful?

A (*Misunderstanding the question*) As far as Karen is concerned, it has given her the opportunity to have a breathing space; it's taken her out of the other situation; it's taken the pressures completely off of her. She doesn't have to think – well, what am I going to do next? She knows she is in for the time being. In the mean time a lot of work has been done with her, I have visited her on several occasions, staff have talked to her at length, she has settled down, she has got stuck into her work.

And was her authorisation justified? Clearly, it was designed to save her from herself, and Karen appears to accept the propriety of this, her hedonism being ultimately destructive. Perhaps, though, the script is not quite so simple, for although Karen appears to be playing the part of the prodigal returned, not only is she doing so in concepts and language which she seems to have acquired from the professionals but she even chose her own audience. Before she agreed to meet the researcher, Karen, who had been described to us by her social worker as 'scheming, a lot of her behaviour was planned', asked for a specified member of staff to sit in on the interview:

Q Do you think you were in moral danger?
A Now I look back I do, but when you are out there you don't. Now I realise that I was, in a way. When I was out there I felt I was my own person. I didn't have to ask anybody what I did. Now, with me being only 15, I shouldn't have done it.
Q Do you think you have been fairly treated or not?
A It's fair being put in care; I was causing a lot of bother at home. It was Mum as well, but I was rebelling back at her. In the end she stopped me going out, so I stopped going to school so that I could go out in the day. I was causing her a lot of bother, 'cause she's got my little sister to look after. So in a way, it was fair . . . . I just need a period to think about it, just to realise what I've done in the past.

Some feminist critics of the juvenile justice system have attacked as heavy-handed paternalism, as evidence of double standards of sex morality, the use of state restrictions on 'wayward' girls (see, for example, Smart 1976; Campbell 1981). Girls, according to this approach, might better be allowed their free sexual expression in a manner more available to boys. Other writers, influenced by recent debates about child sexual abuse, have argued for a more decisive intervention to protect children (especially girls) from sexual encounters to which they are insufficiently mature to give informed consent. Into which of these categories a 15-year-old girl with a disruptive family background, confused and unhappy, who repeatedly absconds from all open situations, who prostitutes herself while on the run and finally asks to be held in security should fall is an interesting question. Karen's image of the secure unit is the idealised one of the home she has never had, the home that makes her *feel* 'secure', which gives her relationships of a non-exploitative kind which she has not previously experienced. It would presumably be difficult to describe these reactions as merely symptoms of institutionalisation, though they do reflect the seventh of the practice dilemmas articulated in the last chapter: 'You can talk to the staff here. The girls are nice. There are proper lessons here. Talking to the staff is the best thing, because you've got to get your problems out anyway.'

Case E: Sarah Holmes

Sarah is a 15-year-old girl with a lengthy history of residential care; her mother is a lesbian prostitute, her father in prison for sexually abusing her, and she herself has, through her parents, a history of involvement in child pornography, as well as offences, over-dosing, solvent abuse and non-school attendance. She was described to us by her unit manager as 'much more sinned against than sinning'. When Sarah last over-dosed, her mother, with whom she has not lived for many years, sat outside the hospital for several days but refused to see her; in an especially poignant paradox her only warm relationship is with her father, who, following his abuse of her is, like her, currently locked up.

Unusually, through a combination of strong solicitor and weak presentation by the local authority, Sarah several times successfully opposed secure accommodation applications. She persistently absconded from open units, however, and was deemed unsuitable for community-based treatment facilities. As a multiple-need child she was beyond the scope of facilities for offenders *or* the psychiatrically disturbed *or* persistent absconders, and no unit could offer her help with all three problems. After periods of psychosis her mental state was now apparently restored to a degree of equilibrium, and she was now considered less in need of psychiatric treatment than psychiatric oversight.

Sarah was a bouncy, hyperactive girl with darting eyes and prone to making sudden physical movements. Her narrative, though in parts confused and confusing, spoke powerfully for itself, not least in relation to her management of her single narratee, whom she clearly saw as someone to whom she wished to make complaints, on whom she wished to create a certain impression, and through whom she wished to impress some of her fellows. What she said may or may not have been true; in her own mind truth and fiction were probably blurred to the point of indistinguishability. As we remarked before, however, even falsehoods can be loquacious. She came into the interview room giggling and glancing behind her, clearly having been discussing her prospective interview with girls who had already been seen and outlining to them what she was going to say. Her voice was noticeably loud:

Q What do you think of the unit?
A I hate it. I think it's stupid. Everyone in there (*pointing*), they said it was fair, but I don't. Don't tell any of the staff I said so.
Q No I won't.
A Well, I hate it, can't stand it. It's unfair and it's stupid. It just is. Right. Do you know much about me?
Q Not very much. Tell me about you.
A (*Describes in detail the various open homes where she has lived, and how she absconded.*) But I never ran away, I just did burglaries. And that was unfair why I came here in the first place. I didn't think it was fair – I couldn't believe it. All right, the police said if I did any more burglaries, which I did, they were going to put me in, you know, secure, but they never. And social services put me in secure for running away, which I never. I never ran away. They gave me a warning. I never ran away again. I did burglaries, that's all. I went out one night and I did them then, oh, and I was 20 minutes late coming in, and I got picked up by the police. They picked me and this lad up – he's much too young, 15. He's really thin and can get in anywhere.
Q Do you like doing burglaries?
A No, I – well I did, I don't know really, because in kids' homes you don't get enough money. You know, when you smoke, it just uses up all your money, and everyone nicks fags off you, and by about Monday, Tuesday you've run out of money, and you have four days to go without fags. That's why people do it. And everyone at that home – they either nicked from shops or they did burglaries. Only a few of them weren't, not many. And the staff there were horrible, really horrible. 'Cause they don't mind you sniffing or anything. Say you were sniffing in your bedroom and wanted something for a headache. All they say is 'you shouldn't sniff then'. They don't mind; they say that they can cope with that but they're stupid – they don't cope with it, they just ignore it.
Q What do you think they ought to do?
A I don't know. In a way I'm pleased that they didn't do anything; it's only now that I'm thinking of them as being uncaring.
Q Do you sniff glue?
A Do I heck! You're joking. You don't get a chance.

Q Do you think you will when you get out?

A Not saying. I might not, but I might. I don't know, I think I might because it's not illegal to sniff, and you can't get put into secure for sniffing can you? That's stupid, that.

Q Only if they think it's putting your health in serious danger.

A Not really. I mean, the most vulnerable to dying through sniffing is in the first couple of months of sniffing, 'cause in the first couple of months your body can't – or you can be knocked out. Because I remember when I ever first sniffed, this lad put half a can in a plastic bag. Now you shouldn't put that much in, and I passed out. If it hadn't been for him I would have died. He had to bang me on the back and all that lark. It's only really bad for kids about 13 or 14, sniffing on the run, and they pass out – they can't help themselves choking.

Q How many children's homes have you been in?

A (*Gives a list*) Some in here have been in twice as many, but social services – I don't know whether I should say it – do a really, really bad job. Because they've never had kids they do what they think is best for us, but they don't know that what they are doing is not best for us. Because locking us up in these places is not fair; it's like a prison sentence. It's not natural. They say it's for your own safety and that lot, but they don't know when someone's locked up all they think about is getting out and doing some damage to somewhere – I'm not saying that I will, but that's all anyone thinks about.

I never got into any trouble at all when I was at home with me dad. I was really, really good. All right, I was sneaking out at night and I was into drugs, but what I am getting at is, the social services didn't know. So as far as they were concerned I was all right and I wasn't in any trouble. I sneaked out and went to night clubs and sold drugs, but they didn't know that then, so that wasn't a reason to take me into care.

Everyone thinks that because I'm locked up in here I'm all right, but that's not the case, is it? I mean everyone says your past is over with, and you can't change it, but I've never been able to cope with my problems, and I need to talk about them, but no one's prepared to listen. How can someone look to the future if they can't live with the past?

(*Describes an episode of absconding*) Did you hear about me on the radio? I was on the radio; they were looking for me. When I got out I thumbed it. I wanted to get to our house so I could get all the tablets. I got a lift with this lad. He said he was going to Wales, so I said I would go with him. But I had to go in our house first to get

> some money and some tablets. I went in, got the money and tablets and went to Wales. I came back. I hated social services, wanted to be in my own bed with my own teddies. I couldn't get back into our house. I went to the next door neighbour and collapsed. I nearly died. Wish I had. But I shouldn't say that because everyone wants me to look positive. I really freaked out. I had tubes everywhere when I woke up. Then I came back here and they said just work the system. Even if you are going to kill yourself don't tell us 'til you get out. In other words don't do it on our territory.
>
> I think it would be best if I went to a place, not a hospital, but a place with a psychiatrist or a psychologist on the premises, and it's a place especially for people who've had child abuse, and assaults and drugs and sniffing. So that everyone could tell about their problems, everyone could understand each other, and everyone could help each other in their own little way.

It would, of course, be difficult if not impossible to place this narrative in the realms of formulaic literature precisely because it presents us with such complex issues. The narrative style itself is internally shifting: the girl actually assumes different *personae* as she proceeds, switching unpredictably and with bewildering rapidity from rebel without a cause, to little girl lost, to victim of a hypocritical and oppressive machine, to someone triumphing over that machine. The fact that Sarah *was* all these things makes it as difficult to place her narrative as it does to deal with her in 'real' terms: she poses a problem which only something as ambiguous as secure accommodation can contain.

That her narrative is peppered with obvious contradictions and, in the midst of a truly tragic tale, intermittent bouts of comedy (not all of which have translated to the printed page) makes it no simpler. The irony operates on at least two levels. First, there are 'obvious' contradictory stories about absconding, drug dealing and burglary which, were this a work of fiction (with the critic thereby able legitimately to suspend human compassion) would make Sarah akin to a comic character from the pen of Dickens or Jane Austen – Sarah Gamp, perhaps, or Mrs Norris from *Mansfield Park*. Secondly, however, the irony exists also in the narrative's original form of oral autobiography, told to a chosen audience of one, who had clearly been 'set up' by the girl as a naïve receptacle for her pathetic (in the Greek sense) bravado. Sarah's transparent 'use' of her audience is clear to us as narratees but not to her as narrator, for almost certainly she does not know that we know that she knows. The gap between her naïve perception and our knowing one is profoundly, and literally, ironic.

CONCLUSION

Five children then, in some ways as different from each other as they could be, in others very similar. All five are outsiders who do not 'fit in' conceptually or administratively, whose circumstances and behaviour have no precise 'name', who have no obvious 'home' other than secure accommodation. The nature of their problems is beyond the explanatory capacity of the professionals, even of those specialist experts whom the professionals consult. This, combined with the fact that their problems also have a strong 'public' dimension and that in a range of ways they will not recite the correct script, playing the willing convalescent, worries the professionals whose restrictive decisions are therefore a product less of the wish to oppress than of concern, confusion, anxiety and weakness. The children are in secure accommodation both because it is a 'somewhere' to contain them *and* because it is the only obvious *locus* in which they can be helped to confront their various difficulties.

Of the boys, Michael's behaviour disturbs because what he will do next is unpredictable, David's because it is all too predictable, while Richard causes concern because no one knows what – if anything – he has actually done. This alone has kept the professionals guessing hard, and notwithstanding their self-restraint in refraining from asking him whether he is guilty as charged, the professionals suspect he is, have uncovered family problems which might help explain his supposed 'actions', and think his parents think he is guilty. Hence they are now considering receiving him into care, a possibility which justifies the quasi-therapeutic work they are doing with him – work precisely characteristic of a secure unit.

Of the girls, Karen's lifestyle has caused concern and raised an awkward question about sex discrimination: does her vulnerability to the power of men justify, even necessitate, a more decisive intervention on the part of the state than would be the case with a boy, or is such an intervention merely a matter of blaming the victim for her own victimisation? Even this difficult question is further complicated by the fact that Karen wishes to stay in the institution which has given her the only home she has known. Where lies the coercion? In locking her up or in ignoring her wish to be locked up?

Sarah's power on the other hand is diffuse, stereotypically 'mad' in its web of both affective and intellectual dislocation and flashes of blinding insight. Yet this is, perhaps, a very comprehensible response to a biography which precisely manifests this dislocation: her mother both visits her in hospital and does not visit her; her father both abuses and loves her; her whole life can only be understood by being viewed through the looking-glass. Her manner, conduct and experiences provide ample material for psychiatric and social diagnoses, but her circumstances, the practical concerns of the social workers, remain desperate, her future bleak and, at age 15, possibly short.

The five youngsters have in common that they are all, for various reasons, to stay in secure accommodation. They have caused public problems in the past, lighting fires, committing indecent assaults, possibly committing a serious crime, being prostitutes, burglars or drug abusers. Their future behaviour is unpredictable not just in the sense that all behaviour *is* unpredictable (MacIntyre 1981: 85) but because the expert explainers seek but cannot find the 'root cause' of the problem. Needs, rights and interests are finely related, as are the duties of the professionals to the children themselves and to those who might be damaged by them if they were released. Hence it is simplistic for the House of Commons Social Services Committee to say 'the care system is designed primarily to provide protection for children against adult society rather than protection for society against children' (House of Commons 1984: xiii), not least because it is impossible to disentangle the two in the day-to-day world of professional decision making. Certainly in the cases of these five children and many more like them, in the absence of secure accommodation it is difficult to see where they would go; the best efforts of the professionals are actually the best efforts of us all to understand, engage and solve the intractable problems they pose, and that the experts are so often unsuccessful is hence no condemnation of them. Their task is not fundamentally curative but a necessary form of action in a society to which the idea of an insoluble problem, a state to be endured, is so alien. In contemporary western society the active pursuit of the impossible is more culturally acceptable than the stoic acceptance of pain, hardship and misfortune.

We have used a literary motif to help us understand something of the children and their situations. Like Gaston Dominici, however, the children are not fictional characters, and to speak of them thus is by no means to demean, trivialise or mock their experiences, some of which are truly horrific. We view the children as we view fictional characters because we use the same spectacles to see the children as we do to read a book. This in turn raises a further question:

> There is a logical puzzle at the heart of the theory of literature. It concerns fictional characters. The puzzle is simply this: What exactly *are* fictional characters? We talk readily and authoritatively of Faustus and Fanny Price, Tom Sawyer and Uncle Toby, and often delight in doing so. Furthermore, we acquire beliefs about them and even argue about their true nature. Yet there are no such people and we know that perfectly well. Is all this talk, then, about *nothing at all*? What is

> fictional, to be sure, cannot be *real* but characters it seems cannot be *nothing*. So what in the world are we talking about?
>
> (Lamarque 1983a: 52)

Lamarque's answer, which seems to us substantially correct, is that fictional characters 'are' a collection of abstract properties and attributes presented in recognisable human form. Our interest in humans, however, is also frequently abstract. Hence, 'our interest in newspaper stories about people unknown to us seems comparable to our interest in fiction. It also explains why fiction can play such a serious and instructive part in our lives' (Lamarque 1983a: 82). And, we might add, why so many of us are devotees of those newspapers and magazines (including – perhaps even especially – satirical magazines) which, by blending 'fact' and 'fiction' into an integrated whole, create an 'art' form transcending the binary divide between them, rendering 'truth' an insignificant determinant of motivation for readership. Perhaps this is what Roland Barthes had in mind when he observed: 'What I claim is to live to the full the contradiction of my time, which may well make sarcasm the condition of truth' (Barthes 1973: 12).

6 Insecure accommodations

The judicial hearings

> Liberal writers . . . invite us to see the Supreme Court's function as that of invoking a set of consistent principles, most and perhaps all of them of moral import, in the light of which particular laws and particular decisions are to be evaluated . . . . But if my argument is correct, one function of the Supreme Court must be to keep the peace between rival social groups adhering to rival and incompatible principles of justice by displaying an even-handedness in its adjudications. So the Supreme Court . . . played the role of a peacemaking or truce-keeping body by negotiating its way through an impasse of conflict, not by invoking our shared moral first principles. For our society as a whole has none.
>
> (MacIntyre 1981: 235–6)

> You can argue your case, but unless the criteria, the body and the bed coincide at the same time, you can't proceed with anything. That is one of the biggest menaces of all. Secure accommodation availability has gone absolutely bonkers.
>
> (Interviewee)

We have described the procedures followed for the court observations in Chapter 4; here we discuss the observations themselves a little more fully. The role and function of the courts emerged as a theme not only in the observations themselves but throughout the study. The juvenile court's intervention shifted the 'meaning' of secure accommodation by emphasising the necessity of protecting children's 'rights' alongside (but not instead of) meeting their needs and interests. This was by no means universally seen as a bad thing: 'She's going to oppose renewal of the order; she's going to fight us tooth and nail, and a little part of me wishes her good luck' (field social worker).

The new legislative restrictions constituted a further stratum in the totality of secure accommodation: the therapeutic freedom of secure units to develop long-term treatment programmes was logically disturbed (though not, as we discovered in our fieldwork, prevented); the relationship between child and professional – or at least the professionals' view of that relationship – was affected by the introduction of the notion of challenge; phased release from absolute security to absolute freedom was no longer possible.

The heterogeneity of the secure accommodation system is such that a strategy which protects children's 'rights' against incarceration in small 'holding' units also affects the capacity of large, sophisticated, highly professional and well-staffed units to complete treatment plans of empirically validated effectiveness, thereby meeting those same children's needs and interests. The legislation poses the problem, insoluble in a juvenile court, of how to protect children against 'bad units' while enabling the work of 'good units' to proceed. To protect children's rights *at the expense of* their needs and interests would, after all, scarcely be a tangible advance; inevitably therefore the role of the courts as protector of 'rights' can, even if that role is played to perfection, supplement but not replace that of the professional decision makers in the local authorities.

JUVENILE COURTS AND WELFARE AGENCIES

The role of juvenile courts was discussed with local authority decision makers in the policy study. Though the legislation introduced a new formal element into the relationship between social services departments and the magistracy, its practical impact on their working relations was slight. Any assumption that the hearings would be topics of keen mutual interest was rapidly dispelled: though in forty-six areas formal meetings with magistrates periodically occurred, only four interviewees reported meeting specifically about secure accommodation; the frequency of meetings varied from more than three-monthly (fifteen cases) to less than annually (eleven cases); interviewees could seldom tell us who attended the meetings; and several interviewees reported magisterial reluctance to attend them, one Bench in particular describing them as 'interference'.

Few had had cause to view the hearings themselves with apprehension: 72 per cent of our interviewees had never experienced an unsuccessful application and 38 per cent had never even experienced an application being contested. Though 86 per cent knew of renewal applications being made, only 12 per cent had heard of one being turned down; only 14 per cent had ever heard of an appeal, and only 4 per cent of a successful one.

Specific courts, particularly those close to a secure unit, had a reputation of being 'tough' because they tended to issue authorisations only after rigorous enquiry, and, knowing this, some respondents, when seeking a renewal of an authorisation, would exercise their right to elect for the case to be heard in the 'home' court, not in the 'tough court' close to the unit. On the whole, however, respondents regarded the most difficult discussions as those which took place within their own departments when the decision to proceed with an application was taken. It was widely held that, as one respondent put it, a combination of weak case, strong solicitor and independent-minded court was necessary for an application to fail.

Informants' opinions of the courts varied, but were predominantly uncomplimentary. The idea of courts protecting children against the misuse of executive power was widely seen as fantastic, and interviewees themselves were quick to blame other local authorities for, as they saw it, misusing their power by exploiting courts' complaisance. For example, one respondent informed us that 40 per cent of all Unruly Certificates issued nationally were issued in his region: 'The East Hillshire figures are good. It's over in West Hillshire that they're very heavy, and that partly seems to be the authorities' attitude, not just the magistrates.'

There was scarcely more confidence in courts' management of applications:

> It's hard to know what magistrates are doing in some quarters. We're very unhappy about practices that we see in other parts of the country. I mean it may be an exaggeration but I'd say that 80 per cent of all court orders that come to us from other authorities – there's something wrong with them.

And in another interchange:

> I don't think they listen to the facts, I just think they will always err on the side of caution, and if there's any doubt at all they just make the order on the ground that the local authority can always bring them out if appropriate.
>
> Q So they make the order and just leave it to the discretion of the authority?
>
> A Yes, though that's only a personal opinion.

Court–agency relations proved fertile ground for anecdotal narrative. In some stories the court fitted easily into the role of the foolish opponent of the wise department:

> With one girl we had an application turned down – the court just offered a shorter term order than we were asking for and we had to go back in and we fought that one and we won the longer term. She had had lots of bits of 72 hours – a very difficult girl – and then we went to court for a 6 month renewal. She was always independently represented, had her own solicitor. Finally after a riot with members of staff seriously injured

> . . . that girl is now in long term security at a YTC. . . . I don't know what it was, maybe the Bench or something. This girl was a high risk, you see.

Other agencies told stories against themselves, describing situations where they were struggling with new roles, grappling with the complexity of managing professional staff in a field where feelings often ran high. In the following account there is a rift between the views of a junior staff member and those of management. Social worker and agencies are following different scripts, and the clash is reflective of the moral incommensurability (MacIntyre 1981: 68) between individual 'rights' and bureaucratic utility to which we have already referred; the result is public fiasco:

> An application was refused and that was really on evidential grounds, because we had a social worker called to give evidence by the boy's solicitor and he was against the application. This was one of the few occasions where things have gone badly wrong beforehand. There had been no proper discussion between the social worker and the secure unit staff, and when it came to court the solicitor picked up that the social worker was actually unhappy about the application and called the social worker to give evidence. And when certain questions were put to him and he answered what was his opinion not what was the departmental view the application was refused. That obviously led to certain procedures being introduced to prevent it happening again.

Overall, respondents' views of the juvenile court were complex and ambivalent. Very few rejected the role of the courts in principle, some expressed relief that 'the buck stopped somewhere else', some developed considerable respect for the more experienced courts, and in particular for some solicitors specialising in child-care cases. On the other hand this approbation seemed dependent on the court's bark being worse than its bite. Few interviewees who had had an application rejected were other than critical.

This criticism is best understood as the first of four main reasons why we believe that any confidence in the court's capacity to protect children from the intervention of an over-zealous executive would be misplaced: as the professionals are explainers, not excusers, their case is based on professional judgement, not instructional relationship. Hence for a court to reject an application is seemingly for a lay Bench to question the competence of a professional, and one with whom they will be working in the future.

Secondly, the contemporary politics of child care make any rejection of applications on the part of courts a high-risk activity. Be the child demonic villain or mucky angel there is a public interest in his fate which is precisely met by the intrinsic ambiguity of secure accommodation: whether the child is threat, victim or both, his being at large causes worry. Though the child's 'nature' may be beyond grasp, his behaviour must be managed, and in a way which reflects the ineffable character of its aetiology.

Thirdly, no one involved in proceedings perceived them as qualitatively distinct from a trial in which the child was defendant and the social services department prosecuting. Authorisations, which specify the maximum period a child may be held and only then while the circumstances which led to the authorisation being made continue to apply, were almost invariably seen as a sentence: like the youngsters themselves, many interviewees referred to children 'getting three months'.

In the large majority of cases where applications were unopposed by the child, consistently with the court's role in a criminal trial but not with the function of a civil liberties tribunal, 'no challenge' was normally taken as equivalent to a 'Guilty' plea. This tendency occasionally took an extreme form. We were told of one boy, Martin Henry, known (but, since his mother refused to attend court, only through hearsay) to be aggressive at home, and who was a persistent absconder from open accommodation, but whose circumstances fell outside the criteria for an authorisation. A senior manager told us:

> His own solicitor and the Guardian [*ad litem*] took the view that his behaviour and lack of parental control were *prima facie* grounds for a secure order. That was not the view I took although I had the most vested interest in obtaining a secure order.
>
> Q His own solicitor felt he should go into secure accommodation?
>
> A Yes. We made considerable efforts to meet this boy's needs through the community, but it was completely unsuccessful. He systematically evaded all attempts to reach him or even speak to him. Secondly we felt there was a strongly collusive element from his mother – though over the last 18 months that has shifted to the boy having a dominant role over the mother. We then tried a residential unit, which was the next increment, and he never stayed on it for more than two hours, and he also failed to appear before the court for a hearing. And at that point we started to look into 21A. We actually looked at the wording of the law and we felt that the child running away and being beyond parental control was not of itself grounds for a secure order: we could not see any evidence that physical, moral or mental welfare would be at risk. I saw the mother a few times with the social worker and said to her 'the only way you will get a secure order is if you stand up in court and say he has been violent to me', and the grandfather stands up and says 'the boy has head-butted me'. In fact the mother declined to do this, and she was under some pressure from me to do this, but she never did. When we

wrote the court report – and it was so controversial it had my signature at the bottom – let me read it to you, shall I?

> It is the intention of the local authority to request a series of interim care orders, perhaps three or four. This will enable us to test out the efficacy or otherwise of a particular pattern of interventions which will be outlined in the conclusion. The first two requests for an interim care order will be accompanied by a request for a secure order under 21A. The request for a secure order is both important and yet controversial . . . . There is no evidence that Martin Henry is in moral danger, a risk to himself or to other people. He is, however, a chronic absconder. We do not believe that a child suffering from Martin Henry's difficulties of being beyond control a priori fit the criteria for a secure order. Further evidence should be required. Nevertheless there is a broader argument and we will request that the court considers it. The welfare interests of the child are clearly not served under present conditions. He is completely beyond any reasonable control or apprehension either by himself or the local authority. . . . If Your Worships are unable to grant the secure order then it is unlikely that any plan of action will succeed, and the local authority will formally withdraw the care proceedings.

The fact that the authorisation was made is the clearest proof yet of two of our arguments: that the wording of legislation is not the main source of action and that a withdrawal strategy is ineffective. No solution other than security appeared to exist, and the local authority manoeuvred events so that the court, if other than compliant, would have to field the consequences in a publicly embarrassing situation. The professionals – social workers, police, justices' clerk, the boy's solicitor – colluded to encourage the magistrates to make a seemingly illegal authorisation on a passive boy because it seemed the only thing to do.

The fourth problem for the court as protector of liberty stems from the interaction of the localised nature of the magisterial system (see, for example, Harris 1992: ch. 7), the infrequency of applications and the lack of magistrates' training in secure accommodation procedures and decision making. Interviewees in both the policy and the background studies stressed the respect they had for some 'experienced' courts, and it was also noticeable that in some courts adjacent to large units there was sufficient work to make specialism in this field a possibility for local solicitors. Accordingly, the standard of argument was high, and not unusually spilt into a second day. Most magistrates, however, deal with few applications, for in the 'heavy user' courts the size of juvenile panels is large and few magistrates hear more than a handful of applications in a year. Variable standards of practice are the price to be paid for all juvenile (or youth) courts being permitted to hear applications.

JUVENILE COURTS AND SECURE ACCOMMODATION APPLICATIONS

In common with most western systems of juvenile justice (see Klein 1984), the English and Welsh system performs a number of functions. From the first it combined civil and criminal jurisdictions which required it to act both as *parens patriae* and as dispenser of justice. The management of juvenile justice increased in complexity with the increasing emphasis given to the welfare of the child between 1933 and 1969, and as we saw in Chapter 1 the two jurisdictions became steadily more blurred.

This blurring did not, however, lead to uniformity, for the ambiguity which we have been describing as an attribute of secure accommodation is the very microcosm of the ambiguity of juvenile justice generally (Harris 1982; Webb and Harris 1984). Accordingly, just as we saw in Chapter 4 the remarkable differences between the attitudes of Agencies C and D to secure accommodation, so in the juvenile justice system there exist extremes of courts dedicated on the one hand to welfare and on the other to punishment (Anderson 1978). For all these variations, however, such evidence as there is about consumers' perceptions of the courts suggests that whatever the court thinks it is doing the children feel themselves on trial (see, for example, Parker *et al.* 1981). The children we interviewed for the criteria study largely endorsed this view.

Undoubtedly, the cognitive as well as procedural shifts necessary to deal with a civil petition, not a criminal hearing, are considerable. It has been argued that courts are better structured to deal with children as threats than with children as victims, and more comfortable doing so (Eekelaar *et al.* 1982). In our study we encountered courts which pressured local authorities to apply for an authorisation, and several situations in which an authorisation was treated as akin to a sentence, with Benches adjusting its length on the basis of mitigation speeches from the child's solicitor. We also learned during the policy study of various 'deals' between courts and local authorities in which authorisations were issued instead of Unruly Certificates on the understanding that the child would not be discharged into open conditions.

In secure accommodation applications the proceedings are, to the uninitiated, similar to those of a criminal trial. The youngster is called on to answer serious (though sometimes non-criminal) allegations, and the fact that the court is there to defend the child's rights against the local authority, not to determine guilt or pass sentence, is a distinction whose subtlety was beyond the comprehension of the children to whom we spoke. Indeed, studies of the magistracy give little reason to see Benches as likely effectively to uphold a civil libertarian function: magistrates are 'decent people picked for their ability to get on with other decent people' (Burney 1979: 212) rather than for mental incisiveness, theoretical expertise or demonstrable commitment to the rights of the individual. Put another way:

> The justice of magistrates' courts is what Weber called Khadi justice, having its own order and rationality but dealing with localized troubles in a way that is consistent with community sentiments and individual circumstances. As such, it does not rest on literal-minded attempts to apply abstract rules so much as an attempt to solve practical social problems by the creative use of those rules.
>
> (Dingwall and Eekelaar 1984: 110)

When we add to this an unavoidable lack of experience in dealing with 21A applications and the fact that discussion about them does not feature large in their meetings with social services departments, we might anticipate an inclination to complaisance with the wishes of the local authority. And so, as we shall see, it transpired.

Applications almost never entail contests over questions of fact; where disputes occur they are normally over interpretation. A child seldom denies having absconded, for example, but there is room for debate as to the point at which a child who has absconded is deemed to have a 'history' of absconding, and hence to become eligible for an authorisation. And these are complex matters of interpretation where courts have little guidance, few ground rules, and this complexity is increased in renewal applications when courts are required to rule whether criteria admitted or proven at the first hearing still apply. This is inevitably difficult and sometimes impossible given that the child will have had little opportunity either to add to an absconding record or to demonstrate a change in behaviour while in secure accommodation. Matters of this kind were seldom aired fully in court, and any standardisation of decision making in these fraught and complex cases was achieved not by the sophisticated application of statute, case law or superior court guidance but by a magisterial preference for endorsing the application.

At the time of our study secure accommodation applications were not covered by the Guardian *ad litem* system; since the implementation of the Children Act 1989, however, non-criminal youngsters have been so covered and it will be important to monitor the impact of this change. When we conducted our fieldwork, no independent assessment of the child's needs, rights and interests was provided, and it was assumed that the care authority's social worker would, without conflict, be both dispassionate expert and 'prosecution' witness. In none of the hearings observed was an independent social worker employed by the child's solicitor, and accordingly the weight of professional 'explanation' rested on the care authority, the social worker's opinion, almost inevitably in favour of secure accommodation, standing also as the *ex cathedra* pronouncement of a professional expert. This seemed to us a point where ambiguity was both unnecessary and unhelpful, and it is to be hoped that the extension of the Guardian system to embrace non-criminal youngsters will go some way towards solving this problem.

A further complication relates to the role of the child's solicitor, and our findings confirm Hilgendorf's view that solicitors' practices vary widely. The advocate

> may present to the court a particular view of the matter, argue for an interpretation of events or seek a given outcome. To do so involves the advocate in decisions about the interpretation of events and judgements about what to do in the best interests of his client . . . . A young child clearly cannot give instructions and there are difficulties about whether an older child can take decisions about what is in his best interests.
>
> (Hilgendorf 1981: 50–1)

In our study it was clear that solicitors also found themselves juggling needs, rights and interests. A solicitor specialising in secure accommodation cases told us:

> Solicitors are frequently asked to oppose applications when there is no real alternative for the child and little opportunity to investigate other possibilities. One is often in the very difficult position of doing what is in the best interests of the child (frequently because they are not capable of giving proper instructions and they have no parents to assist them in so doing) and, on the other hand, opposing an application because one is specifically requested to do so. Invariably to oppose an application is not in the best interests of the child and yet the law gives the child the right to do so.
>
> In most cases the child gets on well with the social worker, but if one is opposing a section 21A application one must consider how far to go in cross-examination. Whatever the outcome, the child will continue to need a social worker if he/she is to obtain the help and support needed. Over-zealous cross-examination could destroy a relationship.

So courts almost never have access to any independent professional assessment of need, in the past at least the care authority acted as party to the proceedings *and* as an agency of professional assessment, and the child is often insufficiently mature or intelligent to give instructions. These problems are exacerbated by the fact that hearings are dealt with by lay Benches, and some solicitors are of the view that eloquence in a weak case may lead to an outcome at once successful for, but detrimental to, the child. In practice this was rare (though not, as the case of Sarah Holmes demonstrates, unknown) and we found disagreements between Benches and social workers to be rare (see also May and Smith 1980: 298). Similarly, 60 per cent of solicitors in Hilgendorf's study were critical of courts' competence:

> They commented that the lay magistracy is not really equipped to deal with the complex legal and psychological issues raised in child care cases and that the bench tends to be overimpressed with the professional expertise of the local authority. They felt that in practice the court acts as a rubber stamp for decisions taken by the local authority.
>
> (Hilgendorf 1981: 135)

That courts almost always endorse the requests of professionals should not surprise us given the ambiguities involved in the nature of secure accommodation, the legally and socially sanctioned role of 'explainer' ascribed to the social workers, the power of the professional in western society, the political 'risks' involved for lay Benches in acting against professional advice in fraught cases, the continuing working relationships between courts and professionals and the courts' lack of experience in dealing with these numerically few applications. Though the high proportion of successful applications is not self-evidently a problem (it may after all simply reflect the soundness of bureau-professional decision making in determining whether to proceed to court), we have already reported a number of concerns which those involved have expressed about courts' competence to do their job.

We have rejected the view that most of the problems can be dealt with by 'tightening' the legislation. Whether a child is to be held in secure accommodation is only in the strictest sense a legal question. More fundamentally, secure accommodation is the solution to an unsolved problem which cannot be ignored. If the legislation is drafted too tightly it will create unintended exclusions, and deviance and collusion will follow, with the 'facts' massaged to mean what they have to mean if security is to be obtained. And, as we have seen, the characteristic of advocacy in this field is that the solicitor may well be a party to this necessary conspiracy to do what, in all the circumstances, seems to the professionals the right thing to do.

The issue is not, therefore, primarily one of legal sophistication, for the nature of social workers' 'expertise' does not, *in ultimo*, lend itself to stringent testing. Where there is an omission, particularly given the subordinate place of knowledge to agency power in local authority social work, is in the absence of any independent social-work scrutiny of applications, and, though time will tell, the Guardian system may go only some way towards addressing this problem. Indeed, if the effect of this extension were to give sovereignty to rights over needs and interests, we might find more children like Sarah Holmes, at physical liberty, but disturbed, unhappy and putting themselves in danger.

Courts can act as formal checks on executive powers. Though they could, given the crucial nature of pre-court discussions, increasingly question local authorities closely about their own pre-court discussions, querying why particular alternative facilities had been rejected, it would be unrealistic to expect such questioning radically to affect the proportion of successful applications. After all, even the 'tough' court already mentioned, though it subjected the professionals to searching scrutiny with hearings frequently running into a second day, relatively seldom rejected applications: in seventy-two cases (sixteen opposed) heard in this court over a 30-month period, only five applications for authorisations were refused.

This may not matter if the court's reputation or conduct promotes closer pre-application consideration by the local authority; and the fact that some local authorities took pains to avoid this particular court suggests that this is indeed a likely consequence. Certainly, for many social workers courts remain daunting places, and it seems desirable for this healthy anxiety to be fostered if the temptation to collusion is to be minimised: 'social workers significantly overestimate the probability of "losing" a case. The few instances where the court overrules their recommendation loom large in their thinking and tend to overshadow the vast majority where the decision is in their favour' (Hilgendorf 1981: 138). We conclude, therefore, that the main value of intensive scrutiny of applications is not primarily that it will lead to increased proportions of rejections (though this may of course be the case) but that it will press the crucial decision makers, the local authorities, both to be cautious about which cases to bring to court and to take steps to develop alternative facilities. Making an application should not be an easy option for local authorities, and while the extension of the Guardian system will make it less easy than it was, there may be scope for making it less easy still. In this the courts do have an important role to play.

THE OBSERVATIONS

Some of the difficulties encountered in managing this phase of the study were described in Chapter 4. Practical considerations aside, however, it quickly became clear that there was little purpose in extending the study to incorporate the eighty hearings originally envisaged. The picture we obtained from observations undertaken in five high-usage courts was of the courts being presented with difficult problems and a clearly recommended course of action by the care authority, with little or no opposition from the child's solicitor. In only one case did the hearing last more than 30 minutes, and the hearings were significantly shorter than the full care hearings whose brevity was itself criticised by Hilgendorf:

> From our observations of juvenile court hearings we believed that in some cases there was reason to doubt that the court was acting as an independent decision-making body. . . 7 of the 33 observed cases took half an hour or less to hear including 2 which took less than 10 minutes.
> (Hilgendorf 1981: 138)

In this section we report briefly the hearings under the main criteria included in our observers' schedule: waiting time, length of hearings, the nature of representation and the decision. The picture overall will be disturbing to many. Hearings seemed to have low priority to the court administrators, with waiting times on average more than five times as long as hearing times. Nevertheless, in a minority of cases 'waiting time', far from being an unnecessary encumbrance, was the time when the hearing was 'fixed' by the professionals. The judicial hearing, already, in our account, less significant than the decision making of the social services department, was further marginalised in at least the few cases where our observers either 'listened in' or spoke informally to the main actors while waiting for the hearing to begin, by 'deals' struck by the professionals to provide the court with an agreed set of arrangements. Whereas in other 'accounts' of court-room drama (Carlen and Powell 1979) the ironic element is that everyone except the defendant knows the script, in these cases the outsiders were the magistrates.

Though most magistrates appeared to have little idea of the complexity of their task (and indeed made their decisions speedily and without *Angst*), solicitors, who clearly were more aware of the distinction between civil petition and criminal trial, were divided as to how best to proceed. We have seen already that taking instructions in child-care cases is not straightforward, and our solicitors adopted either a passive or a bargaining mode. *Passive* solicitors generally supported the local authority's position: some had clearly encouraged their clients not to oppose; some had spoken to the social worker to clarify the longer-term objectives; and some simply felt that secure accommodation was the only realistic response to an otherwise impossible situation. *Bargaining* solicitors transferred their mitigation skills to this arena by 'talking down' the length of authorisation requested by the local authority, but courts' reactions to this approach seemed, as we shall see, unpredictable and by no means always related to the apparent strength of the case.

The problem for the solicitors was, as we shall see, the impossibility of engaging with the discourse of social work from within the discourse of law (for a particular perspective on this problem, see King 1991). The legal discourse has to do with matters of proof, clarity, logic; that of social work with complexity, hypotheses and prediction. In a field such as ours, where the two discourses meet, there is no single way 'through', no correct manner of pronouncing in favour of one and against the other, no obvious strategy of 'integration'. And, in the absence of advice which would corroborate or challenge the social worker's opinions *in their own terms*, it is asking much of the local juvenile court to exercise the wisdom of Solomon when the professionals themselves have seemingly failed to do so.

Waiting time In all five areas the children were produced at the start of the court day. Delays before the hearing were frequently considerable. The observer at Court E was spoken to thus by a disgruntled residential worker:

> It didn't seem like a big list, but they always leave the secure accommodation orders until last, which seems ridiculous to me. When one of these kids goes berserk in the waiting room and hits someone then they'll get their act sorted out.

In this case the boy had waited 119 minutes for a 5-minute hearing at which, since he decided to oppose at the last minute, an interim order was made. The rearranged hearing the following week was the only one observed which began on time (an afternoon court having been set aside for it) and, at 135 minutes, was the single longest hearing observed.

In the five courts the mean waiting time was 93.7 minutes, with a median wait of 100 minutes and a range of 0–206 minutes. In the five individual courts the mean varied from 75 minutes (Court D) to 109.7 minutes (Court B). In only a minority of cases was a reason for the delay given, when it was most frequently the result of the non-availability of a solicitor. These reports give something of the flavour:

> The hearing was very short compared with the time the child had to wait in a closed room. He was brought to court before 10.00 a.m. yet because of another time-consuming case and the movement of solicitors between courts, S's hearing did not take place until two and a half hours later. One of the police had tried to get the hearing put forward without success and also asked the social worker to have a word with the boy. The room in which he was kept was without facilities and interests.
>
> (Case L: waiting time 155 minutes; case 10 minutes)

> The room has no facilities beyond a bench, a wall on which many have written in the past, and a toilet which is kept locked – access is gained

by tapping on the room door to get the key from the policeman who will open the toilet door, or may allow the boy to open it and unlock it himself under supervision.

(Case M: waiting time 75 minutes; case 18 minutes)

Length of hearings The mean length of all hearings was 17.2 minutes, the median 13 minutes (the mean having been inflated by the single 135-minute case), the range was 3–135 minutes and the modal length 15 minutes. Thirty-six of the thirty-seven cases were of 30 minutes' duration or less, and on average youngsters waited five and a half times as long for the case to begin as the case took to hear. Surprisingly, with the exception of the 135-minute case, opposed hearings did not take significantly longer than unopposed ones: the median length of opposed hearings was 15 minutes, against 12 minutes for the unopposed. In eight of the twenty-seven unopposed hearings the length was less than 10 minutes, and in five it was 5 minutes or less.

Observers several times commented on the brevity of the hearings, and it was clear that in some instances by tacit agreement among the professionals part of the court's job – such as explaining the situation to the child in 'ordinary language' – had already been undertaken informally outside the court. In the hearings themselves the children appeared 'outsiders': one observer described the scene in a manner which illustrates just why hearings 'felt' to many of the children like a trial:

> The manner of the magistrates was always calm and polite towards the child, with no hint of a patronising or dominant attitude. Court room was rather large with plush green carpet, curtains and highly polished tables. Magistrates were three in number on a dais, slightly raised. Facing the Bench, solicitors and court officers spoke from the left side and the Clerk from the right. All participants spoke in rather subdued voices. There was noise from a fan and from a few people entering and leaving the court during the proceedings. The magistrate addressed the boy when telling him to remain standing at the start, and when he was told he could sit. Apart from his solicitor the boy had no other support. It was clear that various people had spoken to the boy before the hearing, but no one asked for his opinions during the proceedings.
>
> (Case H)

Representation In all but one case, in which the boy's father had dismissed the boy's solicitor, the youngsters had exercised their right to legal representation. In that case the drama was widely perceived as comic, the comic motif lying, as it does in, for example, *A Midsummer Night's Dream*, in the gap between the importance and complexity of the role and the incompetent manner in which it was performed by a confused and inarticulate outsider:

> Father sacked solicitor shortly before hearing, so there was no legal representation. Father spoke himself and in a convoluted way appeared to be opposing the application. There was a certain amount of amusement on the part of some court officials, and the expectation was there that the father would have his say, but that the local authority would get what it wanted. Boy seemed very isolated, sitting alone in the front row, and almost incidental to what was happening. Everything seemed very 'tied up': the family are well known to social services and courts apparently, and the dismissal of their solicitor appeared to have diminished their case. There did not appear to be much consideration given to what father had to say.
>
> (Case N: length of hearing 25 minutes; result: 6 months secure accommodation authorisation)

Elsewhere representation was variable but predominantly *passive*. In Case W 'the solicitor felt it was futile to oppose the application due to circumstances'; in another 'the solicitor said that he and his client supported the application in view of the care and support at the Unit' (Case Y); in another the solicitor asked the social worker 'if P could be moved to an open unit during the 6 month period. Social worker said it was up to him to behave himself. Solicitor said he agreed and was not opposing' (Case Z11).

In yet another case:

> The solicitor said he had read the social worker's report and was satisfied with it. He was pleased with the improvement D had made and it seemed he now had an aim in life. Though the criteria were frequently stated when the first application was made there was no mention of them during this (renewal) hearing. Also, though the social worker's report was written the magistrates did not take up the court's time to read it. The solicitor did not seek to reduce the authority's request for a 6 month extension; no one asked why D's good progress was not good enough.
>
> (Case K)

Sometimes the solicitor's main job seemed to be outside the court:

> The hearing was very short. I would have expected some attention being paid to what the local authority hoped to achieve in the time. Child's solicitor got up only to say that the application was 'not contested'. The child, one assumes, had spoken with his solicitor but nothing of the interaction emerged in court and no one else spoke on behalf of the child,

or asked the child to speak for himself. Even the fact that the child's moral welfare was at risk was left implicit.

(Case J)

Solicitors who were not passive on a number of occasions performed in *bargaining* mode, conceding that secure accommodation was appropriate but using the techniques of advocacy to minimise the length, albeit with varying degrees of enthusiasm:

> This hearing was for an interim authorisation. It was not opposed but the defence planned to oppose at the full hearing. The defence solicitor at this hearing suggested a 7 day interim order, the local authority asked for 28 days and the order was made for 14 days.
>
> (Case C)

> History of sexual assault, TDA etc. Most recent incident – indecent assault on member of secure unit staff. Defence solicitor queried length of order; after the hearing the social worker told me that the solicitor was trying to get an order for 3 months, but it was not pushed very hard in court. This hearing seemed even shorter than the others I have attended.
>
> (Case Z7; length 7 minutes).

In the following case, by talking informally to the participants during the waiting period, the observer was able to show that the 'real' bargaining was done prior to the hearing:

> Solvent abuse said to be connected with offences. Solicitor asked whether a 3 month order would be sufficient. Social worker would be concerned about this, as it would take a lengthy time to stabilise R's behaviour. R's 18th birthday was in February, so the order would effectively be 5 months. 'Deal' was made by the secure unit staff: when he appears at Crown Court for taking and driving away a motor vehicle they will argue for him to stay at the secure unit for 'treatment' purposes rather than go to youth custody for 6 months; in return he would agree not to oppose the secure order. This is what happened in court.
>
> (Case Z9)

Cross-examination by the child's solicitor occurred in only six cases, in only one of which was the length of authorisation less than that requested. In this case a vigorous set of questions around the notion 'history of absconding' may have led the court to strike a compromise between the two sides, both of whose cases had merit. The argument about the criteria, rather than being determined in favour of one side or the other, was bypassed by an expedient akin to 'passing a lenient sentence', a debate about principle being resolved by a technical device:

> The solicitor argued (on interpretation of criteria) that absconding had taken place over a short period of time. Before this period and since, the boy had cooperated with the authority. He asked whether the boy could be allowed home on trial. Solicitor asked the field social worker if he considered the boy's being behind locked doors and always in the company of a member of staff as punishment. Social worker said he did not. The treatment programme aimed to increase the boy's freedom gradually. The solicitor said the boy perceived that he was being punished and had told him he would not abscond if placed in open accommodation. He pointed out that the written report from the unit demonstrated that the boy had made good progress. The magistrate said nothing except to announce the Bench's decision. No statement was made to give reasons for the fact that it was to renew for only 3 months instead of the 6 requested.
>
> (Case I)

Elsewhere, cross-examination was not successful. In this case the boy had already been in security for 9 months:

> Solicitor questioned whether a second period of 6 months was justified. Social worker explained that P had not settled down at the open unit and had absconded very frequently; at the secure unit he was beginning to make good progress. Apparently to get the social worker to be more explicit about what constituted 'good progress' the solicitor asked whether the boy had been given any treats. The social worker said the boy was not yet allowed off the campus but it was hoped that his freedom might be extended. The solicitor asked whether a review of the situation after 3 months might not be more appropriate. The social worker said that period would not be long enough to achieve the desired progress. The solicitor asked whether the boy was really progressing or whether it was that there was a lack of alternative facilities which could be more appropriate. The social worker stated that the boy was making progress but agreed that there was no other place suitable for carrying out such a treatment programme.
>
> (Case M)

One is reminded of Dworkin's comment:

> The difference between dignity and ruin may turn on a single argument that might not have struck another judge so forcefully, or even the same judge on another day. People often stand to gain or lose more by one judge's nod than they could by any general Act of Congress or Parliament.
>
> (Dworkin 1986: 1)

Representation, in short, is always available, but not only is it variable in quality but the nature of secure accommodation means that it has a less obvious relation to outcome than in a contested criminal trial. It is difficult for a solicitor to penetrate the social worker's 'professional opinion', and the decisions a court can make may be influenced less by the relative force of argument and counter-argument than by the necessity of dealing pragmatically with the problem in front of it. Bearing all this in mind, the most effective part which a solicitor can play may well be in pre-hearing negotiations which enable an agreed proposal to be put to the court. This has the effect of acknowledging that the procedure is what we believe it to be: less a public and libertarian activity of protecting the interests of the powerless individual against the encroachment of the state than a bureaucratic negotiation akin to a case conference, in which everyone is concerned to achieve the least bad outcome in a messy and difficult situation.

The decisions Magistrates had little difficulty in reaching their decision, retiring to consider in only four cases. Authorisations were granted in thirty-two of the thirty-seven cases (all but one for the length of time requested by the authority); four interim authorisations were made; and in one case the application was dismissed, but in interesting circumstances. The child, aged 16, faced numerous criminal charges and had a serious criminal record. His absconding from a remand home led to the present application, which was not opposed:

> The social worker told the court that a report could not be prepared until next week. The court was pushing to sentence him today and the social worker was questioned to this effect. Social worker, brother and solicitor all supported the application but the magistrates felt his bad criminal record of recent offences committed justified their making a remand in custody for a week and not in the local authority secure unit. The lad had been in care since 10 years of age for delinquency, and his care order was revoked recently, so it was felt that social services had reached the stage where they could no longer positively supervise.
>
> (Case V)

This idea that secure accommodation exists in tariff relation to other forms of 'custody' is not unique to the courts: in another instance where an interim authorisation had been sought and granted, a secure unit social worker told our observer that at the full hearing the unit would be 'recommending youth custody – we don't want him back'.

CONCLUSION

It will be clear that the idea that judicial hearings protect the liberty of individuals against excessive state intervention is, so far as secure accommodation is concerned, little more than libertarian rhetoric. With some exceptions the picture is of somewhat desultory hearings, few characterised by serious disagreement, and without any apparent relationship between force of argument and outcome. The court, as the visible tip of an iceberg of bureau-professional decisions and pre-court accommodations, is a decision-making body only in the most formal sense. While the existence of hearings may meet the requirements of the European Convention on Human Rights, local courts are competent to offer neither authoritative interpretations nor consistent applications of law; they can influence only informally the development of the facilities which might obviate the necessity for the applications being made; they cannot effectively interrogate those 'professional judgements' of social workers which, as we have seen, derive less from sound theoretical knowledge than from personal experience or agency policy. Missing from the hearings is any guarantee that this judgement has been challenged on equal terms by another professional.

For these reasons, we doubt that the refinement of legislation will significantly affect court practices. This is not, however, to suggest that nothing can be done to improve the practices of the courts. Closer scrutiny may pay particularly rich dividends in *renewal applications*. We have mentioned that, once in secure accommodation, youngsters tend to stay there: renewal applications are normally rubber-stamped. First, however, the requirement to prove that the original criteria continue to exist is impossible to meet in many cases (one cannot, after all, easily abscond from a secure unit); secondly, some units offer 12-month treatment programmes when the maximum renewal period is 6 months, so creating pressure for further renewal; and thirdly, we have observed a curious internal contradiction that, whereas a child who is not 'responding' can self-evidently not be released, one who is improving sometimes also seems to need to stay longer in order to take more of the successful medicine. This problem emerged repeatedly, and leads us to conclude that to focus less on admission than on discharge might constitute a practical contribution to reducing the population of secure units. The temptation to regard secure accommodation as a 'solution' rather than a temporary opportunity to freeze the child's world while a solution is sought is strong. It may be fostered by a complaisant solicitor and, indeed, the child, for whom, as we have seen, secure accommodation, precisely because it is *not* a prison, can be so very welcoming, homely and, of course, 'secure'. Hence:

The defence solicitor was pleased with progress but did not seek to reduce the authority's request for a 6 month extension, nor did the court officer indicate this as a possibility. No one asked why D's good progress was not enough.

(Case K)

The application was sought in order to continue with a training programme which included education, individual and group counselling. S had told his solicitor that he felt his 6 month stay in security to be quite long enough.

(Case L)

The hearing was very short. I would have expected some attention being paid to what the authority hoped to achieve in the time.

(Case J)

Father challenged the residential social worker to defend the educational provision available to his son, who he was most anxious to see back in mainstream education. The worker stressed the improvement in N in the past 3 months – educational and social needs were being set and developed, and rehabilitation home was envisaged at an appropriate time. Magistrates commented on the good, concise report submitted by the head of unit, also favourably, on the boy's progress, and the value of seeing things through.

(Case N)

C has made good progress at the unit, but the various social services people feel it is too soon to integrate her with other people at the unit.

(Case Q)

Boy was responding very well to treatment; it was now felt that a further order would greatly assist in the treatment. Magistrates commended the boy for his positive response to present treatment, adding that it would be expected that after these next 3 months he could be trusted to return to the open unit.

(Case Y)

During the social worker's evidence the magistrates at first seemed to be questioning the few incidents he had detailed, but then the slant seemed to change and they asked whether 3 months was long enough to do the work necessary to move her out of the secure unit.

(Case Z6)

So good progress is insufficient to justify discharge from secure accommodation, as are conformity and obedience, which, as David Harding discovered, may be interpreted as a form of manipulation that, far from demonstrating progress, conversely 'proves' its absence. The nature of secure accommodation makes it difficult if not impossible to measure progress except in relation to the norms of the unit itself, adherence to which has little predictive potency precisely because it may well indicate not repentance or reform but merely that the child, in order to be freed, is willing and able to play by the unit's rules.

The danger of being 'lost' in secure accommodation exists, and the courts – and particularly children's solicitors – have a part to play in interrogating social workers at renewal hearings not only about the *child's* progress but also about *their* progress in developing and implementing a non-secure strategy. For the 'problem' presented by secure accommodation may be less about admission than discharge. At a certain point the child ceases to be one for whom secure accommodation is a passing exigency and becomes one for whom it is the preferred mode of long-term treatment. The 6-month renewal period is in some respects the worst of all possible worlds: long enough for the 'passing exigency' child to slip down the social workers' list of priorities and imperceptibly become a 'long-term case' but not long enough to provide the permanence, asylum even, which a truly damaged or damaging child may require when discharge is impossible.

It may be that the involvement of the Guardian *ad litem* will reduce this problem. Certainly the work of the courts would much benefit from the greater use of independent social work reports at renewal as well as initial hearings – for enquiries into the competence of social work cannot be effectively undertaken by lawyers and magistrates alone. While this would not of itself 'solve' the problems identified, it might reduce the scope for the professional response to these dilemmas of wishing them away and so failing to act decisively. Statutory reviews of children in secure accommodation do not invariably have the sense of urgency which the intensity of the intervention demands, and while the reasons for this hesitancy will by now be clear, it is not for the professionals to regard ambiguity as justifying inaction. For in yet another paradox, inaction is itself an action as indecisiveness is a decision, and, in the case of secure accommodation, action of an especially decisive kind.

It is not enough, therefore, to accept secure accommodation as the 'somewhere, something' or the 'black hole' depicted in this book. To refer to secure accommodation as ambiguous is not to deny the possibility, indeed the urgent necessity, of professionals developing clear lines of action in a particular 'case'. That such clarity is not simple to attain we do not doubt, and our encounters with Michael, David, Richard, Karen and Sarah stand testimony to this difficulty. Yet all these children will at some point be disgorged into the world where their problems lie, and in our study it was not always clear when and why the decision to discharge would be taken or, to reiterate our repeated question about David Harding, what they would have to do to get out. In that process the court, though it cannot be central, yet has an important part to play, but one which it is not presently playing to the full.

7 What is to be done?

> To be human and to be aware is to encounter only what is in some manner understood. Thus, it may be said that understanding is an unsought condition; we inexorably inhabit a world of intelligibles. But understanding as an engagement is an exertion; it is the resolve to inhabit an ever more intelligible, or an ever less mysterious world. The unconditional engagement of understanding I shall call 'theorizing'. It is an engagement to abate mystery rather than to achieve definitive understanding.
>
> (Oakeshott 1975: 1)

> Humanism and technocracy, individual interest and social utility, rights and virtue, therapy and punishment, and rehabilitation and deterrence – the fixed positions in these debates are not simply to be shuffled into a duality which gives primacy to the individual on one side and the order on the other. Each possesses the potential to be deployed on behalf of a politics of order; the rhetorical and organizational resources of one become available for use when those of the other fall short of the mark.
>
> (Connolly 1988: 70–1)

Our journey has sought to take us, by a somewhat complex theoretical route, towards the abatement of mystery, though undertaking it was also a prerequisite for perceiving just how deep and diverse the mystery was. We began by describing the form and context of secure accommodation which, we showed, exists as a small but vital cog in the much larger wheel of the relations of state, family and child. This relation is multifaceted, reflected in civil and criminal law and in public, and in particular social, policy; and it is varied over time and place. From a broad historical perspective the state, as it has expanded its legal code and welfare provisions, has moved away from a night watchman role towards one based on a more decisive form of collective responsibility. As this role has developed, the provision of goods and services and the imposition of control over those who receive them have become both inevitable and inextricable. From this has emerged a particular, but perpetually mutable form of social contract.

The policies of public child care form, alongside a variety of other services ranging from transport policy to health care, from policing to customs and excise, an aspect of this relationship, and hence of the social contract. Public child care in particular has attributes which make it especially important: the intervention of the state in family life which it entails both signifies and constitutes changes in the nature of the state itself, in the rights and duties of the family and in the idea of childhood. We saw historically, in our consideration of Ariès, that while the state has become more interventive (and the family more private) neither state nor family has entirely divested itself of its former trappings. Hence, alongside the contemporary view that the state should, for example, protect abused children or enforce certain standards of parent-craft, there exists another view that for the state to do *too* much of this points to totalitarianism and the attenuation of individual responsibility. These themes constitute the warp and woof of much social policy (Harris 1990), and the pathway between them is steered by professionals making strategic decisions, reacting speedily to problems, 'balancing' a move in this direction with a gesture in that, but fundamentally accommodating both forms of political belief in their work. Neither of these themes (nor any of the 'value perspectives' enunciated by Lorraine Harding) makes sense alone, however, for they are but ideal types of merely analytic and heuristic utility, and to adhere to any one at the expense of any other would constitute an impossible, unthinkable rigidity.

In child-care practice, therefore, the professionals accommodate conflicting views stemming from accumulated historical strains which are inextricably part of our own cultural settlement. We do not protect children at the cost of destroying the family any more than we prevent road deaths at the cost of abolishing the motor car. We try, always, to ensure that the cure is not worse than the disease: whereas in road safety we make laws, vary penalties, experiment with different enforcement patterns, embark on advertising campaigns, lecture schoolchildren and improve training, in child protection we try to prevent abuse and to identify and help abused children, but only while maintaining the power of the very parents who, statistically, present the greatest risk of abuse itself.

These perpetual processes, however, imperceptibly but inexorably change the social contract between state and family and indeed the nature of state and family themselves. As our view of childhood divests itself increasingly of the trappings of paternal property, the state inevitably assumes new duties. The question *quis custodiet ipsos custodes*? is, in child care, answered clearly: professionals, particularly social workers, police the parents, but only to a degree and when there is reason to do so. When they fail to do enough or, conversely, when they overstep the mark, complaints, scandals, campaigns and enquiries ensue, before a new equilibrium is established with new laws, procedures, training. Though professionals may complain about the supposed injustice of this, what is sought of them is precisely *not* rigid adherence to an impossible ideal based on a single 'value perspective' but the sensible and mature accommodation of necessarily conflicting principles. There is no crude Laingian 'double bind' in this, any more than there is in the action of the parent in telling the quiet child to speak up and the noisy one to calm down. In all these forms of human relation it is the golden mean which is sought, a mode of behaviour containing the right blend of humours to be culturally appropriate.

As the contemporary view of 'the child' shifts in the direction of what is best termed 'limited citizenship', the child's relation with the family must shift too. In this sense the notion of a family holding the child in 'trust' (Dingwall *et al.* 1983; Dingwall and Eekelaar 1984: 106–11) is perhaps the subtlest expression of a complex situation. Children's law constitutes the terms of the trust, and to breach it is, therefore, to breach the trust itself, so surrendering the rights of trusteeship. Children lack full citizenship 'rights' because they lack the capacity to exercise them maturely (Freeman 1983; Franklin 1986), but they acquire other rights, with concomitant duties, stemming from that very immaturity. Children have the 'right' to be protected from harm and the 'right' to education and certain additional resources which they may from time to time require; they also have the 'duty' to go to school, to keep the law, to refrain from certain activities permitted when performed by adults. Such variations in 'adult' rights and duties are deemed both socially desirable and in children's own long-term interests, interests of which it is also deemed that they themselves are frequently not the best judges.

As 'childhood' has increasingly come to be viewed thus, the accretion of attributes which characterise 'the child' has become more complex. The simple divide between the needs of the child and the crimes of the adult has been bridged by the concept 'delinquency', a necessary but awkward amalgam of the child with unmet needs and neglected interests who has *also* behaved unacceptably. It is when this 'bundle' of concepts is both at its most inextricable and its most pressing that secure accommodation emerges as a response.

If secure accommodation is not 'just' a prison and not 'just' a hospital provided by a benign and altruistic state, it becomes necessary to create an intellectual and conceptual tool by which to make sense of its amalgam of functions. This pressing need caused us to reject the more conventional analytic approach of 'breaking down' a social phenomenon into its component parts, seeking instead an interpretive mode which addressed the totality. In doing so, a logical place to begin was with the professionals, asking how they themselves made sense of a phenomenon which existed as a slightly disturbing last resort for their most difficult cases. We were from the first struck by their use of narrative: they made sense of their professional lives less by theoretical exegesis than by telling stories, and as they told them it emerged just how 'dramatic' the stories sometimes were, and how very apposite this was given the dramatic attributes of the job itself.

The stories were not simple, and part of the cross the professionals bear is that they play the opposite role to the normal one of the professional in western industrial society. Far from solving problems easily, making the complex simple and manageable, they uncover multiple layers of complexity, discovering 'causes' for forms of behaviour more easily processed without these interpretations: if *tout comprendre, c'est tout pardonner*, it is better not to understand if we are disinclined to forgive. Social professionals turn simple tales of good and evil, misfortune and oppression, into source material for moral and practical dilemmas which many would prefer not to face.

Narrators are not necessarily 'outside' the events they are portraying, and our narrators were central to the drama: as interpreters, explainers, strategists, they made a particular form of sense of the otherwise incomprehensible, both to themselves and to a wide variety of actual or potential narratees, including the children and their families, other professionals, their own managers, members of the public, friends and relatives, the press, the court and, of course, researchers like us. Like any narrative, the stories we heard were incomplete and tailored to meet the needs of the narrator in communicating an image to a given narratee. This we termed 'presentation', with the same tale having entirely different inflexions in tea-room chat and court report. This phenomenon caused us to remark that to seek the 'heart' of the matter would be quite wrong, for in the social world such a 'heart', 'basis', 'centre', 'core', 'key' or even 'root cause' seldom exists, and the literally unending pursuit of it simply impedes the mature response.

The children too told us their stories, and we showed from the amalgam of tales we heard from both professionals and youngsters that secure accommodation defied encapsulation, being used variously at different times and in different places. The children we met all differed too, sometimes radically, in circumstance and behaviour: secure accommodation is, after all, the 'somewhere, something' needed to hold children who, diverse in needs and behaviour, have in common only that they 'fit' nowhere else. It is in the nature of secure accommodation to catch the uncatchable; in this sense just 'tightening the law' or otherwise restricting usage will merely ensure that the same children surface elsewhere in the system, the challenges they pose unsolved, their situations unchanged. After all, the courts were markedly uninterested in textual analysis or fine interpretation, the youngsters were disinclined to appeal, and any conceivable new wording would still potentially embrace far more youngsters than are the subjects of applications. Secure accommodation is a necessary response to otherwise insoluble problems.

These complexities surfaced again when we considered the court hearings. Introduced as a check on professional discretion (Davis 1971), the courts transpired seldom to perform their tasks in the intended manner. Courts' performance (which was frequently unimpressive) was less important than their existence and the impact this sometimes had on bureaucratic decision making. Few courts had the intellect, confidence, experience, knowledge or will to gainsay the professionals; they received no independent social work advice, nor did they have access to the alternative facilities which we argued were so important a part of effective gatekeeping. As we saw in the case of Martin Henry, even where the law did not permit an authorisation, one could be made in the absence of opposition and the interests of common sense. Tighter legislation alone would create more Martin Henrys.

So what is to be done? It might be thought by professionals and reformers reading this that our analysis has been predominantly gloomy, implying that little if anything *can* be done. This would, however, be a misreading. Though it is true that in this field a simple answer is often a simplistic answer, we have not sought to suggest that history itself is the product of impersonal forces abstracted from the world of political will and action. People, of course, create history, people make changes, people initiate reforms, and in the case of secure accommodation there are certain things which people can do. They are small and gradualist rather than revolutionary, but may help us use secure accommodation in a manner which, while retaining its necessary catholicity, contains its oppressive potential. Some of these suggestions have been made directly in the text, others are implicit in it but are made here for the first time. They are fewer and less detailed than those included in our research report: not only is this book written for a different purpose, but time has passed, legislation has been amended and the Children Act 1989, representing a significant further shift in the overall relations of state, family and child, has been implemented, but not for long enough for us fully to grasp it.

SECURE ACCOMMODATION: SOME POSSIBLE WAYS FORWARD

First, it does not follow from the argument that secure accommodation has about it a necessary ambiguity that it is never misused or that it cannot and should not on occasion be avoided. The youngsters in our study were heterogeneous, containing some whom all but the most fanatical abolitionist would agree should be held for their own good and others who were merely petty nuisances or social casualties with a predilection for absconding from open conditions. We have also seen that the courts' consideration of these matters was generally cursory, and argued that for effective scrutiny to take place it had to be undertaken by someone with direct access to alternative resources and with a continuing interest in the case. Weak gatekeeping is poor gatekeeping, for restricting and rationing are less effective in any problem-solving activity than creating sensible, flexible and practical alternatives.

The case of Martin Henry both made this point and turned it on its head: the court was in effect warned that if it failed to cooperate and make an authorisation which was arguably not legally justified it would be held publicly accountable for the fate of a boy whose behaviour gave genuine cause for concern. Its cooperation under this form of professional pressure demonstrates the impact of such continuing responsibility on decision making, but also gives a hint of a possible alternative way forward. A cash-limited child-care budget is soon exhausted by secure placements, and the incentive to prevent or abbreviate them is therefore considerable so long as the decision maker has this form of professional and financial responsibility. It follows that if local authorities wish to minimise their use of secure accommodation they should ensure that strong gatekeeping responsibility lies with a senior professional in such a position, and that if government wishcs thcm to do so it should concentrate its inspections on gatekeeping policies and practices.

Secondly, however, for justice to be seen to be done these internal processes need bolstering by an independent element throughout the decision-making process. We gave considerable attention in our research report (though not in this book) to the role of the 'independent person' whom, under regulation, local authorities are required to appoint to review the holding of children in secure accommodation after 1 month and then at 3-monthly intervals. We believe that this post needs both defining and strengthening. 'Independence' itself was variably interpreted, the task of the independent person is vaguely couched, the qualities, character and expertise of the person are not cited and the person is appointed, trained and if necessary paid by the very authority whose practices are to be scrutinised.

This does seem a rather qualified concept of independence. Our view is that the independent person should, like the Guardian *ad litem*, be appointed by the court from an approved list, paid from central funds, trained and supported. There is also good reason to consider whether the 'independent person' should be the same individual as the independent social worker mentioned in the next suggestion as likely to prove a necessary aid to the court in determining both initial placement and, in particular, renewals.

Thirdly, we have identified practices in the judicial hearings which will disturb many but, perhaps, surprise fewer. It might be thought that our criticisms of magistrates – and by implication their clerks – have been overly acerbic, for their task is an impossible one, their function being to perform a constitutional nicety rather than to act effectively. Hence, untrained in this field, with little discussion about the issues having taken place with the local authorities, little or no superior court guidance, little idea of what alternatives to secure accommodation do or could exist, and with so few applications to deal with that each one entails *ab initio* coaching from the clerk, the justices can only get by as best they can. And when in the majority of cases no one objects strongly to the making of an authorisation, what are the magistrates to do other than comply?

The constitutional safeguard enshrined in Article 5.4 of the European Convention on Human Rights serves better as a statement of base-line liberty for individuals in an emerging nation without strong democratic traditions than as a helpful way forward in the child-care policies of an advanced democracy. If the courts are to be more effective in checking the local authorities they require access to as much expertise as the local authorities, knowledge of what alternative facilities exist and a detailed account of why they are unsuitable. If government wishes to give teeth to its watchdog, it must specify by regulation that an independent social work report be obtained in all cases and that the local authority be required to identify and collect information about the resources a child in secure accommodation would have needed to remain at liberty. This information might then form the basis of policy development inspections by the social services inspectorate, in order to ascertain to what extent the local authorities are responding to the existence of unmet needs among the children they are looking after. This suggestion goes considerably further than the inclusion of non-criminal children in secure accommodation within the Guardian *ad litem* system.

Fourthly, there is the matter of magisterial expertise. If hearings are to be effective they must be regionalised and conducted only by trained and selected magistrates. Perhaps, given our particular concern about renewal applications, this regionalisation might concentrate on magistrates whose divisions include a secure unit – the very magistrates from whom, we learned, some care authorities strategically remove cases (a power which we take to be in need of urgent reconsideration). No-contest cases present a particular problem, for they are characteristically deemed akin to 'Guilty' pleas, yet precisely because secure accommodation *is* often made so welcoming for children whose other relationships have been cruel, unstable or exploitative they may well wish to stay, thereby sentencing *themselves* to secure accommodation, unwittingly colluding with anxious court and dilatory social worker to ensure that they stay within the system.

Fifthly, we have argued that the 6-month renewal offers the worst of all possible worlds. It (literally) locks in the system the child for whom the field social worker should be actively pressing for alternatives, yet destabilises the child whose stay is unavoidably long term. Our preference is that in the case of a child for whom permanency in secure accommodation is not envisaged, renewals should, preferably by regulation but alternatively by self-denying ordinance of courts and local authorities, normally be of no more than 1 month's duration. This would restrict the use of 6-month authorisations to cases where there was serious and demonstrable risk to self or others, and we suggest restricting it, again by self-denying ordinance in the first instance but we hope subsequently by regulation, to cases where the child has a place on a named educational or treatment programme and formally requests the authorisation. The numbers of children involved would be governed by the numbers of available places on long-term programmes, the facility would be available only in large and well-equipped units, courts would demand firm evidence of violent or self-abusive behaviour, and a formal request from the child (as opposed to tacit acceptance) would be necessary. We envisage such a facility also encouraging phased discharge: the ambiguity of current discharge arrangements has much concerned unit managers who, in our view rightly, seldom wish to disgorge children suddenly into open conditions.

It follows that while we believe that the capacity of youth courts to check the discretion of local authorities is circumscribed, they do have the power to structure their own discretion as to the length of authorisation they will grant (Davis 1971: ch. IV). At renewal hearings 6-month authorisations are easily, even cavalierly, given, and in some cases this has delayed decisions which could have been made more quickly. We were certainly struck, in David Harding's case, by the leisurely manner in which alternative therapeutic possibilities, some quite distant, were being visited by the social worker and by the lack of pressure exerted to proceed with dispatch. If, as we hope following the publication of this book, more meetings take place between social services staff and magistrates, we suggest they negotiate ground rules for the length of initial authorisation to be sought and granted, and for the circumstances in which renewal applications should be entertained.

We urge solicitors not to hesitate to cross-examine social workers, and to bargain down the length of authorisation where long-term holding is not obviously necessary. We hope also that government will continue to review legislation and regulation to ensure that children are not staying unnecessarily long in secure accommodation.

Sixthly, training emerged as a key issue. A recent official report (Utting 1991) also emphasises the role of training, but its tendency to treat the problems of residential child care in terms of individual inadequacy, even pathology, and its consequent failure to address the contextual dimensions we have sought to delineate in this book prevent it from constituting a strong foundation for any training initiative.

We argued in Chapter 4 that secure unit staff were 'in' secure accommodation too, and that the very characteristics of that facility designed to keep children 'in' contributed to the marginal position of unit staff in their own departments. This, added to the tradition of paying low salaries to residential staff, the unsocial hours and the nature of the task itself have combined to create problems of staff morale and competence. Yet secure units depend above all on the quality of staffing because, once walls, doors and keys are in place, secure accommodation *is* the staff. Our picture of secure accommodation is of a facility profoundly complex and ambiguous; yet we know too that residential care generally is a site of periodic but unremitting crisis, danger and abuse of power. Secure units deal with the most difficult and disturbed youngsters in residential care, and aspire to do so based on principles 'other than' those of the prison. Yet the gap between this aspiration and the reality of many of the units we visited was stark. Such units were staffed by hard-pressed, unqualified, untrained and frequently unsupported personnel whose ideas about the importance of 'relationships', of providing 'security', of encouraging youngsters 'not to run away from their problems' were often sensitive and perceptive, yet who seldom knew how in practice to translate them into effective behaviour change.

It is of course personal qualities such as these which humanise the institution and which would, for smaller 'holding' establishments, be sufficient if youngsters' stays there were not on occasion so lengthy. Therapeutic aspirations can, in such situations, actually get in the way, as staff struggle to identify the 'root cause' of the problem, to establish 'what makes this boy or that girl tick', so engaging in a hunt with no quarry, in the vain pursuit of a non-existent and logocentric concept whose main consequence is ever longer periods of incarceration, ever more fantastic therapeutic endeavours. Appreciation of this point is central to the 'competency-based' training needs of staff precisely because it helps determine the nature and character of 'competence' itself: a purely technical or mechanistic approach to the matter will seriously damage the children's health. In Oakeshott's words, none the less relevant for all that they were not written about social work:

> Again, professional education is coming more and more to be regarded as the acquisition of a technique, something that can be done through the post, with the result that we may look forward to a time when the professions will be stocked with clever men, but men whose skill is limited and who have never had a proper opportunity of learning the *nuances* which compose the tradition and standard of behaviour which belong to a great profession.
>
> (Oakeshott 1962: 34)

Unit staff are especially influential in the matter which concerns us greatly of how children, whose continuing problems and imperfections are manifest, are discharged from security. The children's problems are frequently not of a kind which involves pinpointing and dealing with a 'root cause'. Each discovery of each new problem provokes further enquiry and the discovery of yet more problems. When the child trustingly tells the worker all, responding to an adult as she never has before, what could be more logical than that the sense of 'security' which provoked the confidences should be perpetuated? From the fact that it is good for the child and provides satisfaction for the professional it is tempting to create a logic of carceral prolongation, holding for just a little longer the improving as well as the unresponsive child. In a culture whose popular literature is full of magical transformations of evil into good and sadness into joy, hopes and expectations are ever in danger of lacking realism; and also in the worker's mind is the fact that when a risk is taken and a child discharged early, the worker who recommends discharge is unlikely to be able to count on public sympathy and support if things go wrong. What better combination of reasons could one conceive of for deferring discharge for just a little longer?

Seventh, we are naturally aware of the intense pressure to increase the number of secure places, but urge caution in succumbing to it if the danger of repeating the unplanned and unintended expansion of the 1970s is to be avoided. We have argued that:

- legislative refinements alone cannot restrict usage;
- there are many children in respect of whom secure accommodation could be used but who are not currently the subject of applications;
- the most potent predictor of the high usage of secure accommodation is a local authority's possession of a secure unit;
- it is incorrect to perceive the balance of need and resource in simple

mechanical terms: resource is not simply a response to need but also its creator;

- there is no 'type' of secure-unit child who can be identified by professional knowledge, and any increase in places will simply attract more youngsters;
- additional places must and will be filled, else budgets will go into deficit, unit costs increase, political questions be asked and staff jobs be jeopardised;
- the very characteristics of secure units which make them 'other than' prison, and indeed the only 'secure' home some of their residents have ever had, make expansion especially easy and likely to be unopposed by the youngsters themselves;
- the existence of more and hence 'easier' secure places may demotivate authorities in their efforts to produce creative alternatives or improve the quality of their open establishments.

There is no doubt from our research that in some authorities the factor which tipped the balance between a placement in open and secure accommodation was not the single difference of the key that turns, but the more general gap between poorly staffed, under-resourced, questionably competent open establishments and a well-resourced secure unit absorbing the funding which would otherwise have been allocated elsewhere. It was precisely this point that led Karen Jarvis in particular to reject the open unit and, by 'creating' unacceptable behaviour, to manipulate herself into secure accommodation.

Eighth, the use of secure accommodation is less effectively controlled by judicial hearings than by shortage of places. This, however, clearly leads to undesirable forms of crisis management and arbitrariness in admissions. We studied the admission process in our research and uncovered a state of near anarchy. Characteristically, social workers spent many hours telephoning secure units in pursuit of a bed, and unit staff similarly spent many hours saying they were full. At the very least, therefore, we hope that the moves towards developing an improved administrative system will continue in order to increase the effectiveness, efficiency and economy of this process and perhaps permit more rational judgements to be made by unit staff as to whom, on a given day, they will admit.

JOURNEY'S END

> When the future is uncertain the mind turns naturally to the certainties of the past, and finds comfort in what is beyond the peril of change . . . . I wanted the sense of continuity, the assurance that our contemporary

> blunders were endemic in human nature, that our new fads were very ancient heresies, that beloved things which were threatened had rocked not less heavily in the past.
>
> (Buchan 1940: 182–3)

> If we ever succeeded in eliminating all juvenile crime, it would mean that 100 per cent of all crime was being committed by adults; which would really be something to worry about.
>
> (C.H. Rolph, cited in Morris and Hawkins 1970: 154)

Our Prologue began by explaining that our particular approach to secure accommodation would take us on a seemingly circuitous route into the realms of both literary and social theory, but that the necessity of taking such a route would ultimately become clear. Now that we are in what is in effect but not name an Epilogue, we can only hope we have been true to our word, and that the journey has not been without interest and value.

Behind much of what we have argued has been the idea that in the social world things are seldom what they seem, that our best attempts at creating change frequently go wrong in practice and sometimes indeed often rebound spectacularly, often on those least able to bear the consequences – the poor, the deviant and the powerless. This means that to offer simple ways forward in a complex and ambiguous situation cannot always work: for not only is this 'situation' actually a different situation in, say, Workington and Winchester, or Norwich and Newcastle, but the situation in these towns and cities is itself ever shifting, in part as a result of the very social interventions we have been describing. It follows from our analysis that any suggestions we make are broadly conceived and dependent on the motivation and ability of the various professionals and courts involved to monitor their progress, make them work for as long as they are useful and, when their utility has been outlived, discard them, replacing them with whatever has become necessary to make good the damage they will by then have started to do.

The problems with which secure accommodation has to deal are not new, nor is the idea of secure accommodation: prisons, reformatories, industrial schools, the workhouse all had attributes of 'security', all of them performed some of secure accommodation's tasks. Secure accommodation, however, as we have tried to show, constitutes a particular conjunction of the therapeutic and the penal which necessitates rejecting the ideal type explanations of both positivists and retributivists but, because their ideas have been so incorporated into our cultural and intellectual heritage, necessarily containing elements of both, bound inexorably and inextricably together.

It is 'delinquency' which secure accommodation addresses, this complex state in which mischance and naughtiness are simultaneously present. For the state to engage with delinquency beyond the confines and approaches of the criminal law is to posit a certain characteristic of the state as well as a certain understanding of the task of the family and the nature of childhood. Such a conjunction of characteristics and expectations would be impossible in a different kind of society, one lacking either the necessity of state intervention brought about by the individualistic conditions of advanced industrial capitalism (Bellah *et al.* 1985) or the possibility of it, brought about by economic growth and the mature cultural development necessary for the flourishing of liberal values. This cumulative cultural process makes decisive social action especially difficult at those points where differing cultural strands are most closely and inextricably interwoven, and secure accommodation is one such point. Ironically, however, it is where decisive action is most difficult that it is often most necessary, and, as we have shown throughout, this is no less true with our subject than with other points of intra-cultural conflict.

In such a system unbreakable or definitive rules are insufficient. Rules are, however, crucial as guideline and bottom line. As such they can specify the completely impermissible and indicate the general directions in which the professionals must move. This is what government has sought to do in the legislative change with which we have been concerned. By analysing that change historically, theoretically and empirically we have sought to show the complexity and ambiguity embedded in the phenomenon of secure accommodation itself. And it is on those most concerned with the system – unit staff certainly, but especially unit children – that the consequences of this complexity and ambiguity are most decisively visited. This book has sought both to reflect that reality and to suggest certain ways in which to proceed if the weight of the problems is not to become unbearable.

Appendix A

Child Care Act 1980, section 21A

1 Subject to the following provisions of this section, a child in the care of a local authority may not be placed, and, if placed, may not be kept, in accommodation provided for the purpose of restricting liberty unless it appears

(a) that –

(i) he has a history of absconding and is likely to abscond from any other description of accommodation; and

(ii) if he absconds, it is likely that his physical, mental or moral welfare will be at risk; or

(b) that if he is kept in any other description of accommodation he is likely to injure himself or other persons.

2 The Secretary of State may by regulations –

(a) specify –

(i) a maximum period beyond which a child may not be kept in such accommodation without the authority of a juvenile court; and

(ii) a maximum period for which a juvenile court may authorise a child to be kept in such accommodation;

(b) empower a juvenile court from time to time to authorise a child to be kept in such accommodation for such further period as the regulations may specify; and

(c) provide that applications to a juvenile court under this section shall be made by local authorities.

3 It shall be the duty of a juvenile court before which a child is brought by virtue of this section to determine whether any relevant criteria for keeping a child in accommodation provided for the purpose of restricting liberty are satisfied in his case; and if a court determines that any such criteria are satisfied,

it shall make an order authorising the child to be kept in such accommodation and specifying the maximum period for which he may be so kept.

4 On any adjournment of a hearing under subsection (3) above a juvenile court may make an interim order permitting the child to be kept during the period of the adjournment in accommodation provided for the purpose of restricting liberty.

5 An appeal shall lie to the Crown Court from a decision of a juvenile court under this section.

6 A juvenile court shall not exercise the powers conferred by this section in respect of a child who is not legally represented in that court unless either –

(a) he applied for legal aid and the application was refused on the ground that it did not appear his means were such that he required assistance; or
(b) having been informed of his right to apply for legal aid and had the opportunity to do so, he refused or failed to apply.

7 The Secretary of State may by regulations provide –

(a) that this section shall or shall not apply to any description of children specified in the regulations;
(b) that this section shall have effect in relation to children of a description specified in the regulations subject to such modifications as may be so specified;
(c) that such other provisions as may be so specified shall have effect for the purpose of determining whether a child of a description specified in the regulations may be placed or kept in accommodation provided for the purpose of restricting liberty.

8 The giving of an authorisation under this section shall not prejudice any power of any court in England and Wales or Scotland to give directions relating to the child to whom the authorisation relates.

Appendix B

Children Act 1989, section 25

1 Subject to the following provisions of this section, a child who is being looked after by a local authority may not be placed, and, if placed, may not be kept, in accommodation provided for the purpose of restricting liberty ('secure accommodation') unless it appears –

(a) that –

(i) he has a history of absconding and is likely to abscond from any other description of accommodation; and

(ii) if he absconds, he is likely to suffer significant harm; or

(b) that if he is kept in any other description of accommodation he is likely to injure himself or other persons.

2 The Secretary of State may by regulations –

(a) specify a maximum period –

(i) beyond which a child may not be kept in such accommodation without the authority of the court; and

(ii) for which the court may authorise a child to be kept in secure accommodation;

(b) empower the court from time to time to authorise a child to be kept in secure accommodation for such further period as the regulations may specify; and

(c) provide that applications to the court under this section shall be made by local authorities.

3 It shall be the duty of a court hearing an application under this section to determine whether any relevant criteria for keeping a child in secure accommodation are satisfied in his case.

4 If a court determines that any such criteria are satisfied, it shall make an order authorising the child to be kept in secure accommodation and specifying the maximum period for which he may be so kept.

5 On any adjournment of the hearing of an application under this section, a court may make an interim order permitting the child to be kept during the period of the adjournment in secure accommodation.

6 No court shall exercise the powers conferred by this section in respect of a child who is not legally represented in that court unless, having been informed of his right to apply for legal aid and having had the opportunity to do so, he refused or failed to apply.

7 The Secretary of State may by regulations provide that –

(a) this section shall or shall not apply to any description of children specified in the regulations;
(b) this section shall have effect in relation to children of a description specified in the regulations subject to such modifications as may be so specified;
(c) such other provisions as may be so specified shall have effect for the purpose of determining whether a child of a description specified in the regulations may be placed or kept in secure accommodation.

8 The giving of an authorisation under this section shall not prejudice any power of any court in England and Wales or Scotland to give directions relating to the child to whom the authorisation relates.

9 This section is subject to section 20(8).

Appendix C

Extract from the Criminal Justice Act 1991, section 60

1 For section 23 of the 1969 Act there shall be substituted the following section –

23 – 1 Where –

(a) a court remands a child or young person charged with or convicted of one or more offences or commits him for trial or sentence; and

(b) he is not released on bail,

the remand or committal shall be to local authority accommodation; and in the following provisions of this section, any reference (however expressed) to a remand shall be construed as including a reference to a committal.

2 A court remanding a person to local authority accommodation shall designate the local authority who are to receive him; and that authority shall be –

(a) in the case of a person who is being looked after by a local authority, that authority; and

(b) in any other case, the local authority in whose area it appears to the court that he resides or the offence or one of the offences was committed.

3 Where a person is remanded to local authority accommodation, it shall be lawful for any person acting on behalf of the designated authority to detain him.

4 Subject to subsection 5 below, a court remanding a person to local authority accommodation may, after consultation with the designated authority, require that authority to comply with a security requirement, that is to say, a requirement that the person in question be placed and kept in secure accommodation.

5 A court shall not impose a security requirement except in respect of a young person who has attained the age of fifteen, and then only if –

(a) he is charged with or has been convicted of a violent or sexual offence, or an offence punishable in the case of an adult with imprisonment for a term of fourteen years or more; or
(b) he has a recent history of absconding while remanded to local authority accommodation, and is charged with or has been convicted of an imprisonable offence alleged or found to have been committed while he was so remanded,

and (in either case) the court is of opinion that only such a requirement would be adequate to protect the public from serious harm from him.

6 Where a court imposes a security requirement in respect of a person, it shall be its duty –

(a) to state in open court that it is of such opinion as is mentioned in subsection 5 above; and
(b) to explain to him in open court and in ordinary language why it is of that opinion;

and a magistrates' court shall cause a reason stated by it under paragraph (b) above to be specified in the warrant of commitment and to be entered in the register.

Notes

PROLOGUE

1 Here and elsewhere, our use of the concept 'ideology' follows Oakeshott's formulation that it is no part of the practical activity of politics, but rather signifies the general beliefs which might relevantly be involved in the justification of any given political action. In this sense, 'ideology' is a specific form of discourse connected to politics, yet not *of* politics *per se* (Oakeshott 1980). For a somewhat similar conclusion from a decidedly different premiss, see Terry Eagleton's definition of ideology as 'the ways in which what we say and believe connects with the power-structure and power-relations of the society we live in' (Eagleton 1983: 14; see also Eagleton 1991).

2 We use 'narrative' in Genette's sense of 'someone recounting something: the act of narrating taken in itself' (Genette 1980: 26; though for a slightly variant approach, see Chatman 1975). It is crucial to distinguish the act of telling (the narrative, which may or may not be accurate, complete or truthful and which could always have been 'done' differently) from the events being described (the story, or *histoire*). Needless to say, the same 'story' narrated by different people, or by the same person at different times or to different audiences, may be entirely different.

3 We use this word in Barthes's sense as 'a type of speech, everything can be a myth provided it is conveyed by a discourse. . . . Every object in the world can pass from a closed, silent existence to an oral state, open to appropriation by society' (Barthes 1973: 117). To regard history as 'fact' is to mythologise, in that a simple facticity implausibly denies the dimensions of selection which underpin any history – dimensions which are invariably culturally explicable. In this sense 'everything', including 'nature' is history, but history, because its roots are in culture, cannot be 'natural'. For a fuller explication of this point, see Barthes's essays 'The *Blue Guide*' and 'The great family of man' in the same collection.

1 SECURE ACCOMMODATION OUTLINED

1 'Children' is used in this book to include people up to the age of 18. For our purposes the distinction between 'children' and 'young persons' is seldom important, and 'children' and 'youngster' in particular are used synonymously.

2 Or, since the implementation of the Children Act 1989, children being looked after by a local authority.

3 Remands to local authority accommodation with a security requirement may now be made 'after consultation with the designated authority' under the Criminal Justice Act 1991 s. 60. See Appendix C.

4 This formulation is altered in the Children Act 1989 to read 'likely to suffer significant harm' (Children Act 1989 s. 25(1)(ii)).

5 Because these systems are administratively divided between different Departments of State and, hence, different local officials, it does not follow that they are conceptually or theoretically divisible, and we shall, except where there is good reason not to, refer to them jointly as the carceral system. We use 'carceral' to imply a system of general control and socialisation, not merely that part of it which takes place in institutions (i.e. as *in*-carceration). We are, in this, following Foucault's usage (Foucault 1977) but, in that we are not necessarily accepting his evident distaste for such a system, we are using the concept 'carceral' as an analytic but not a moral category, neutral not pejorative.

6 The adjective is not, of course, without its irony; nor is the association of keylessness with openness without its significance.

7 It should, however, be noted that this flexibility is not inevitable. In some Australian states, for example, the preference in both the criminal and the welfare spheres is for more tightly worded legislation backed by *ad hoc* legislation to deal with the unusual problems presented by hard cases. In the Victorian legislature, for example, the Community Protection Act 1990 and the Community Protection (Amendment) Act 1991, widely known as the Garry David (or Garry Webb) Act, were passed to ensure the prolonged imprisonment of Webb, a still dangerous offender who had completed his sentence for attempted murder. This involves the decision on the hard case being made by the legislature; in the UK system it is characteristically made by the executive. Such an *ad hoc* system, though possibly attractive to justice theorists, would be unlikely to be feasible in Britain given the centralised parliamentary system and the already overcrowded parliamentary timetable.

2 THE STATE, THE FAMILY AND THE CHILD: A THEORETICAL ANALYSIS

1 In this book we use 'discourse' in a particular, Foucauldian way, to embrace not only the shared *language* of a particular society, but also the beliefs, assumptions and values of which the language is the 'public' representation. 'Discourse' thus represents the 'rules' by which we 'understand' and 'experience' the social formation. We do not, of course, make the naïve assumption that any 'discourse' is universal, or that there are not multitudinous oppositions, conflicts and misunderstandings within a given discourse. Indeed to Foucault, to whom knowledge (often sustained by language) 'is' power, the reverse is naturally the case.

2 A fuller explication of this point may be found in the works of structuralist anthropologists (particularly Radcliffe-Brown and Lévi-Strauss) and linguists (Saussure and his followers); in those of post-structuralist philosophers and critics, notably Foucault and Derrida (for a helpful account of the debate between Foucault and Derrida on the logical impossibility of Foucault's

argument [Foucault 1971] that madness could be 'comprehended' by means of the oppressive language of the very 'reason' which had itself 'created' madness, see Boyne 1990); and of those moral philosophers who have shown that social and family relationships are part of our own substance, 'not characteristics that belong to human beings accidentally, to be stripped away in order to discover "the real me" ' (MacIntyre 1981: 32; see also Wicker 1975: ch. 2).

3 For a fuller discussion of what he terms 'situational propriety' and 'impropriety', see Goffman 1963.

3 YOUNG DEVILS . . . OR ANGELS WITH DIRTY FACES?

1 Roger Bullock, personal communication.

2 For a helpful account of the debate between Lacanian psychoanalysts and ego-psychologists on this controversy, see Harland 1987: ch. 3; for an account of the related debate between the early Foucault and Derrida, see Boyne 1990: *passim.*

3 A personal narrative from one of us is that the recollection of (a) sitting in a court as a student for the first time; (b) observing a defendant in the dock; and (c) having him produced in the cells for an interview in the space of an hour evoked an almost overwhelming sense of 'going backstage' to meet the actor and wondering what he would be 'like' in 'real life'. It is unlikely that this sense is unique: for an interesting analysis of this very point, see Carlen 1976; Carlen and Powell 1979.

4 See in particular 'The typology of detective fiction' in Todorov 1977; for a more general discussion, see Selden 1985: 56–61. That Propp's morphological study was of the formulaic folk tale is also significant, though for an 'exploratory' attempt to apply morphological techniques to classics as well (including *Middlemarch* and *Phèdre*) see Holloway 1979.

5 Though for an alternative view as to the rigidity of this convention, see Fokkema and Kunne-Ibsch 1977: 28.

6 The point has its literary counterpart in epistolary novels such as *Clarissa* (Richardson 1747/48) and in multiply narrated texts of which a recent example is *Talking It Over* (Barnes 1991).

7 In yet a further layer of textual irony, the French translation of Lodge's book *Small World*, a satire on international academic conferences, implicitly, and presumably unconsciously, reflects its own title and theme by sporting a laudatory Preface by Umberto Eco.

8 Doubtless the analogy with Barthes's black soldier will be self-evident.

9 For a brilliant and relevant exposition of *The French Lieutenant's Woman*, see Hutcheon 1984: 57–70.

10 We use 'tabloid' as a conventional metonymy, for clearly size of the paper does not determine quality of product. The advent, in the late 1980s, of the *Sunday Sport*, however, containing entirely fictitious stories and pictures (including, in one issue, a 'picture' of the gates of Heaven) constitutes a perfect instance of the fusion of fiction and reality. The *Sunday Sport* is precisely 'trash', a collection of popular, not to say salacious, short stories presented in a format conventionally considered to tell 'the truth'. And doubtless in its pages 'truth' and 'fiction' are sometimes interchangeable.

11 For a fuller analysis of narrative as power, and one addressed specifically to social workers, see Rees 1991: chs 3–4.

4 TALKING TO THE EXPERTS

1 Though it is noteworthy that respondents used almost identical phrases about secure accommodation itself in respect of children whom they were anxious to maintain in 'open' conditions.

2 It was extended still further by the Criminal Justice Act 1991, section 64, which stipulates that section 53(2)

> shall have effect, in relation to a person who has attained the age of 16, as if the reference to any offence punishable in the case of an adult with imprisonment for 14 years or more . . . included a reference to an offence under section 14 of the Sexual Offences Act 1956 (indecent assault on a woman).

This offence is currently punishable by only 2 years' imprisonment in the case of an adult.

3 In the third area our interviews have been supplemented by data kindly supplied by Mary Henkel, of the Centre for the Evaluation of Public Policy and Practice, Brunel University, from an Economic and Social Research Council funded study fully reported in Henkel 1991a: ch. 7.

4 Though only part of the reason. For a helpful brief account of Ricoeur's distinction between speech and writing as 'alternative and equally fundamental modes of the realisation of discourse', see Thompson 1981: 51–3.

5 A question in our interview schedule which asked decision makers to compare a child in secure accommodation with another child on their caseload who was not, in order that we might isolate the variables which most powerfully influenced admission, failed entirely.

5 SECURE CHILDREN?

1 All names and potential identifiers have been changed.

Bibliography

OFFICIAL REPORTS AND PUBLICATIONS (COMMAND PAPERS)

Report of the Departmental Committee on Prisons (1895) (Gladstone Report) C7702.

Report of the Departmental Committee on Reformatory and Industrial Schools (1896) C8204.

Report of the Departmental Committee on the Treatment of Young Offenders (1927) (Salmon Report) Cmd 2831.

Report of the Care of Children Committee (1946) (Curtis Report) Cmd 6922.

Report of the Committee to Review Punishments in Prisons, Borstals, Approved Schools and Remand Homes (1951) (Franklin Report) Cmd 8256.

Report of the Enquiry into the Disturbances at Carlton School in August 1959 (1959) (Durand Report) Cmd 369.

Report of the Home Office Working Party on Closed and Other Special Facilities in Approved Schools (1960).

BOOKS AND ARTICLES

Ackroyd, P. (1990) *Dickens*. London: Sinclair-Stevenson.

Althusser, L. (1971) *Lenin and Philosophy and Other Essays* (trans. B. Brewster). New York: Monthly Review Press.

American Friends Service Committee (1971) *Struggle for Justice: a Report on Crime and Punishment in America*. New York: Hill & Wang.

Anderson, R. (1978) *Representation in the Juvenile Court*. London: Routledge & Kegan Paul.

Ariès, P. (1960) *L'Enfant et la vie familiale sous l'Ancien Régime*. Paris: Librairie Plon.

—— (1962) *Centuries of Childhood* (trans. R. Baldick). London: Jonathan Cape.

Bailey, V. (1987) *Delinquency and Citizenship: Reclaiming the Young Offender, 1914-1948*. Oxford: The Clarendon Press.

Barker, F., Hulme, P., Iverson, M. and Loxley, D. (eds) (1983) *The Politics of Theory: Proceedings of the Essex Conference on the Sociology of Literature, July 1982*. Colchester: University of Essex.

Barnes, J. (1984) *Flaubert's Parrot*. London: Jonathan Cape.

—— (1991) *Talking It Over*. London: Jonathan Cape.

Barthes, R. (1973) *Mythologies* (originally published 1957 and trans. A. Lavers). London: Paladin Books.

—— (1975) 'An introduction to the structural analysis of narrative', *New Literary History* VI: 237–72.

Bellah, R., Madsen, R., Sullivan, W., Swidler, A. and Tipton, S. (1985) *Habits of the Heart: Individualism and Commitment in American Life*. Berkeley: University of California Press.

Bennett, A. (1901) *Fame and Fiction*. London: Grant Richards.

Bennett, J. (1981) *Oral History and Delinquency: the Rhetoric of Criminology*. Chicago: University of Chicago Press.

Benton, T. (1982) 'Realism, power and objective interests', in K. Graham (ed.), *Contemporary Political Philosophy: Radical Studies*. Cambridge: Cambridge University Press.

Blumenthal, G. (1985) *Development of Secure Units in Child Care*. Aldershot: Gower Press.

Boas, G. (1966) *The Cult of Childhood*. Studies of the Warburg Institute, vol. 29. London: The Warburg Institute.

Bochel, D. (1976) *Probation and After-Care: Its Development in England and Wales*. Edinburgh: Scottish Academic Press.

Booth, W. (1961) *The Rhetoric of Fiction*. Chicago: University of Chicago Press.

Boyne, R. (1990) *Foucault and Derrida: the Other Side of Reason*. London: Unwin Hyman.

Buchan, J. (1940) *Memory Hold-the-Door*. London: Hodder & Stoughton.

Bullock, R., Hosie, K., Little, M. and Millham, S. (1990) 'Secure accommodation for very difficult adolescents: some recent research findings', *Journal of Adolescence* 13: 205–16.

Burney, E. (1979) *JP: Magistrate, Court and Community*. London: Hutchinson.

Campbell, A. (1981) *Girl Delinquents*. Oxford: Basil Blackwell.

Campbell, T. (1983) *The Left and Rights: a Conceptual Analysis of the Idea of Socialist Rights*. London: Routledge & Kegan Paul.

Carlebach, J. (1970) *Caring for Children in Trouble*. London: Routledge & Kegan Paul.

Carlen, P. (1976) *Magistrates' Justice*. London: Martin Robertson.

Carlen, P. and Powell, M. (1979) 'Professionals in the magistrates' courts: the courtroom lore of probation officers and social workers', in H. Parker (ed.), *Social Work and the Courts*. London: Edward Arnold.

Carpenter, M. (1851) *Reformatory Schools for the Children of the Perishing and the Dangerous Classes, and for Juvenile Offenders*. London: C. Gilpin.

Cawson, P. and Martell, M. (1979) *Children Referred to Closed Units*, Department of Health and Social Security Statistics and Research Division, Research Report No. 5. London: HMSO.

Chatman, S. (1975) 'Towards a theory of narrative', *New Literary History* VI: 295–318.

Children's Legal Centre (1982) *Locked Up in Care: a Report on the Use of Secure Accommodation for Young People in Care*. London: Children's Legal Centre.

—— (1983) *Restricting the Liberty of Children in Care: Guidance on the New Laws*. London: Children's Legal Centre.

Clarke, R. and Martin, D. (1971) *Absconding from Approved Schools*, Home Office Research Unit Report. London: HMSO.

Clarke Hall, W. (1926) *Children's Courts*. London: C. Gilpin.

Cohen, S. (1985) *Visions of Social Control: Crime, Punishment and Classification*. Cambridge: Polity Press.

Connolly, W. (1988) *Political Theory and Modernity*. Oxford: Basil Blackwell.

Connor, S. (1989) *Postmodernist Culture: an Introduction to Theories of the Contemporary*. Oxford: Basil Blackwell.

Davis, K. (1971) *Discretionary Justice: a Preliminary Inquiry*. Chicago: University of Illinois Press.

Day, S. (1858) *Juvenile Crime: Its Causes, Character and Cure*. London: J.F. Hope.

deMause, L. (ed.) (1976) *The History of Childhood: the Evolution of Parent–Child Relationships as a Factor in History*. London: Souvenir Press.

Department of Health and Social Security (1972) *Community Homes Regulations 1972* (Circular LAC 18/72). London: DHSS.

—— (1975) *Secure Accommodation in Community Homes* (Circular LAC 75/1). London: DHSS.

—— (1979) *Inspection of Secure Accommodation for Children and Young Persons: Guidance for Social Work Services* (Kahan Report). London: DHSS.

—— (1981a) *Legal and Professional Aspects of the Use of Secure Accommodation for Children in Care*. Report of a DHSS Internal Working Party. London: DHSS.

—— (1981b) *Offending by Young People: a Survey of Trends*. London: HMSO.

—— (1986) *Children Accommodated in Secure Units During the Year Ending 31 March 1986, England* (A/F 86/21). London: DHSS.

Derrida, J. (1976) *Of Grammatology* (trans. G. Spivak). Baltimore: Johns Hopkins University Press.

Dingwall, R. and Eekelaar, J. (1984) 'Rethinking child protection', in M. Freeman (ed.), *The State, the Law, and the Family: Critical Perspectives*. London: Tavistock Publications in association with Sweet & Maxwell.

Dingwall, R., Eekelaar, J. and Murray, T. (1983) *The Protection of Children: State Intervention and Family Life*. Oxford: Basil Blackwell.

Docherty, T. (1987) *On Modern Authority: the Theory and Condition of Writing: 1500 to the Present Day*. Brighton: Harvester Press.

Donzelot, J. (1980) *The Policing of Families: Welfare Versus the State*. London: Hutchinson.

—— (1984) *L'Invention du social*. Paris: Fayard.

Dreyfus, H. and Rabinow, P. (1982) *Michel Foucault: Beyond Structuralism and Hermeneutics*. Chicago: University of Chicago Press.

Dworkin, R. (1986) *Law's Empire*. London: Fontana Press.

Eagleton, T. (1983) *Literary Theory: an Introduction*. Oxford: Basil Blackwell.

—— (1991) *Ideology: an Introduction*. London: Verso.

Eco, U. (1979) *The Role of the Reader: Explorations in the Semiotics of Texts*. Bloomington: Indiana University Press.

—— (1989) *Foucault's Pendulum* (trans. W. Weaver). London: Secker & Warburg.

Eekelaar, J. (1991) 'Parental responsibility: state of nature or nature of the state?', *Journal of Social Welfare and Family Law* 1: 37–50.

Eekelaar, J., Dingwall, R. and Murray, T. (1982) 'Victims or threats? Children in care proceedings', *Journal of Social Welfare Law* (March): 68–82.

Eliot, T.S. (1919) 'Tradition and the original talent', reprinted in T.S. Eliot (1932) *Selected Essays*. London: Faber & Faber.

England, H. (1986) *Social Work as Art*. London: Allen & Unwin.

Eribon, D. (1991) *Michel Foucault (1926-1984)* (2nd edn). Paris: Flammarion.

Fiedler, L. (1971) 'Cross that border – close that gap', in *The Collected Essays of Leslie Fiedler*, vol. II. New York: Stein & Day.

Fitzgerald, R. (ed.) (1977) *Human Needs and Policies*. New South Wales: Pergamon.

Flew, A. (1981) *The Politics of Procrustes*. London: Temple Smith.

Fokkema, D. and Kunne-Ibsch, E. (1977) *Theories of Literature in the Twentieth Century: Structuralism, Marxism, Aesthetics of Reception, Semiotics*. London: C. Hurst.

Foucault, M. (1971) *Madness and Civilization: a History of Insanity in the Age of Reason* (trans. R. Howard). London: Tavistock Publications.

—— (1977) *Discipline and Punish: the Birth of the Prison* (trans. A. Sheridan). Harmondsworth: Allen Lane.

Fowler, B. (1991) *The Alienated Reader: Women and Romantic Literature in the Twentieth Century*. Hemel Hempstead: Harvester Wheatsheaf.

Fowles, J. (1969) *The French Lieutenant's Woman*. London: Jonathan Cape.

Franklin, B. (ed.) (1986) *The Rights of Children*. Oxford: Basil Blackwell.

Fraser, N. (1989) 'Talking about needs: interpretative contexts as political conflicts in welfare-state societies', *Ethics* 99: 291–313.

Freeman, M. (1983) *The Rights and Wrongs of Children*. London: Frances Pinter.

—— (ed.) (1984) *The State, the Law, and the Family: Critical Perspectives*. London: Tavistock Publications in association with Sweet & Maxwell.

Frost, N. and Stein, M. (1989) *The Politics of Child Welfare: Inequality, Power and Change*. Hemel Hempstead: Harvester Wheatsheaf.

Genette, G. (1980) *Narrative Discourse* (trans. J.E. Lewin). Oxford: Basil Blackwell.

Gewirth, A. (1982) *Human Rights: Essays on Justification and Application*. Chicago: University of Chicago Press.

Glouberman, S. (1990) *Keepers: Inside Stories from Total Institutions*. London: King Edward's Hospital Fund for London.

Godsland, J. and Fielding, N. (1985) 'Young persons convicted of grave crimes: the 1933 Children and Young Persons Act (s. 53) and its effect upon children's rights', *Howard Journal of Criminal Justice* 24: 282–97.

Goffman, E. (1963) *Behavior in Public Places: Notes on the Social Organization of Gatherings*. New York: Free Press.

—— (1968) *Stigma: Notes on the Management of Spoiled Identity*. Harmondsworth: Penguin Books.

Graham, K. (ed.) (1982) *Contemporary Political Philosophy: Radical Studies*. Cambridge: Cambridge University Press.

Griffin, J. (1986) *Well-Being: Its Meaning, Measurement and Moral Importance*. Oxford: Oxford University Press.

Haimes, E. and Timms, N. (1985) *Adoption, Identity and Social Policy: the Search for Distant Relatives*. Aldershot: Gower.

Hardiker, P., Exton, K. and Barker, M. (1991) *Policies and Practices in Preventive Child Care*. Aldershot: Avebury.

Harding, L. (1991) *Perspectives in Child Care Policy*. London: Longman.

Harland, R. (1987) *Superstructuralism: the Philosophy of Structuralism and Post-structuralism*. London: Methuen.

Harris, J. (1982) 'The political status of children', in K. Graham (ed.), *Contemporary Political Philosophy: Radical Studies*. Cambridge: Cambridge University Press.

Harris, R. (1982) 'Institutionalized ambivalence: social work and the Children and Young Persons Act 1969', *British Journal of Social Work* 12: 247–63.

—— (1989) 'Suffer the children: the family, the state and the social worker', Inaugural Lecture, University of Hull. Hull: Hull University Press.

—— (1990) 'A matter of balance: power and resistance in child protection policy', *Journal of Social Welfare Law* 5: 332–40.

—— (1991) 'The life and death of the Care Order (Criminal)', *British Journal of Social Work* 21: 1–19.

—— (1992) *Crime, Criminal Justice and the Probation Service.* London: Routledge.

Harris, R. and Timms, N. (1988) *Between Hospital and Prison or Thereabouts.* Unpublished Research Report to the Department of Health and Social Security.

Harris, R. and Webb, D. (1987) *Welfare, Power and Juvenile Justice: the Social Control of Delinquent Youth.* London: Tavistock Publications.

Hawkins, H. (1990) *Classics and Trash: Traditions and Taboos in High Literature and Popular Modern Genres.* Hemel Hempstead: Harvester Wheatsheaf.

Henkel, M. (1991a) *Government, Evaluation and Change.* London: Jessica Kingsley.

—— (1991b) 'The new "evaluative state" ', *Public Administration* 69: 121–36.

Heywood, J. (1978) *Children in Care: the Development of the Service for the Deprived Child* (3rd edn). London: Routledge & Kegan Paul.

Hilgendorf, L. (1981) *Social Workers and Solicitors in Child Care Cases.* London: HMSO.

Hoghughi, M. (ed.) (1984) *Restricting Children's Liberty: Proceedings of a Colloquium of Section 21A.* Aycliffe Studies of Problem Children. Aycliffe School: Aycliffe, Co. Durham. Mimeograph.

Hoghughi, P., Jenkins, A. and Wilkinson, P. (with Catty, J. and Hoghughi, M.) (n.d.) *Placing Children in Security: the Product and the Process.* Aycliffe Studies of Problem Children. Aycliffe School: Aycliffe, Co. Durham. Mimeograph.

Hohfeld, W. (1923) *Fundamental Legal Conceptions as Applied in Judicial Reasoning and Other Legal Essays.* New Haven: Yale University Press.

Holloway, J. (1979) *Narrative and Structure: Exploratory Essays.* Cambridge: Cambridge University Press.

Holt, J. (1975) *Escape from Childhood.* Harmondsworth: Penguin Books.

Home Office (1960) *Report of the Home Office Working Party on Approved Schools.* HH1014/60R. London: Home Office.

House of Commons (1975) *Eleventh Report from the Expenditure Committee: the Children and Young Persons Act 1969.* London: HMSO.

—— (1984) *Second Report from the Social Services Committee, Session 1983/4: Children in Care*, vol. 1. London: HMSO.

Husserl, E. (1970) *Logical Investigations* (originally published 1928). London: Routledge & Kegan Paul.

Hutcheon, L. (1984) *Narcissistic Narrative: the Metafictional Paradox.* New York: Methuen.

Irvine, E. (1982) 'The Clayhangers: father and son', *British Journal of Social Work* 12: 77–90.

Jones, P. (1989) 'Re-examining rights', *British Journal of Political Science* 19: 69–96.

King, M. (1991) 'Child welfare within law: the emergence of a hybrid discourse', *Journal of Law and Society* 18: 303–23.

Klein, M. (ed.) (1984) *Western Systems of Juvenile Justice*. Beverly Hills: Sage.
Kleinig, J. (1978) 'Crime and the concept of harm', *American Philosophical Quarterly* 15: 27–36.
Lamarque, P. (1983a) 'Fiction and reality', in P. Lamarque (ed.), *Philosophy and Fiction: Essays in Literary Aesthetics*. Aberdeen: Aberdeen University Press.
—— (ed.) (1983b) *Philosophy and Fiction: Essays in Literary Aesthetics*. Aberdeen: Aberdeen University Press.
Levy, A. and Kahan, B. (1991) *The Pindown Experience and the Protection of Children*. Stoke on Trent: Staffordshire County Council.
Lovell, T. (1983) 'Writing like a woman: a question of politics', in F. Barker, P. Hulme, M. Iverson and D. Loxley (eds), *The Politics of Theory: Proceedings of the Essex Conference on the Sociology of Literature, July 1982*. Colchester: University of Essex.
MacIntyre, A. (1981) *After Virtue: a Study in Moral Theory*. London: Duckworth.
Manton, J. (1976) *Mary Carpenter and the Children of the Streets*. London: Heinemann Educational Books.
Maxwell, R. (1956) *Borstal and Better: a Life Story*. London: Hollis & Carter.
May, D. and Smith, G. (1980) 'Gentlemen versus Players: lay–professional relations in the administration of juvenile justice', *British Journal of Social Work* 10: 293–316.
Meyer, P. (1983) *The Child and the State: the Intervention of the State in Family Life* (trans, J. Ennew and J. Lloyd). Cambridge and Paris: Cambridge University Press and Editions de la Maison des Sciences de l'Homme.
Millham, S., Bullock, R. and Cherrett, P. (1975) *After Grace – Teeth*. London: Human Context Books.
Millham, S., Bullock, R. and Hosie, K. (1978) *Locking Up Children: Secure Provision Within the Child-Care System*. Farnborough: Saxon House.
Moi, T. (1985) *Sexual/Textual Politics: Feminist Literary Theory*. London: Methuen.
Morris, A., Giller, H., Szwed, E. and Geach, H. (1980) *Justice for Children*. London: Macmillan.
Morris, C. (1975) *Literature and the Social Worker*. London: Library Association.
Morris, N. and Hawkins, G. (1970) *The Honest Politician's Guide to Crime Control*. Chicago: University of Chicago Press.
Narayan, K. (1989) *Storytellers, Saints, and Scoundrels*. Philadelphia: University of Pennsylvania Press.
Oakeshott, M. (1933) *Experience and Its Modes*. Cambridge: Cambridge University Press.
—— (1962) *Rationalism and Politics*. London: Methuen.
—— (1975) *On Human Conduct*. Oxford: The Clarendon Press.
—— (1980) *The Form of Ideology* (ed. D.J. Manning). London: Allen & Unwin.
Packman, J. (1981) *The Child's Generation: Child Care Policy in Britain* (2nd edn). Oxford: Basil Blackwell and Martin Robertson.
Page, L. (1936) *Justice of the Peace*. London: Faber & Faber.
Page, R. and Clark, G. (eds) (1977) *Who Cares? Young People in Care Speak Out*. London: National Children's Bureau.
Parker, H. (ed.) (1979) *Social Work and the Courts*. London: Edward Arnold.
Parker, H., Casburn, M. and Turnbull, D. (1981) *Receiving Juvenile Justice: Adolescents and State Care and Control*. Oxford: Basil Blackwell.
Parton, N. (1985) *The Politics of Child Abuse*. London: Macmillan Education.

—— (1991) *Governing the Family: Child Care, Child Protection and the State*. London: Macmillan Education.

Penz, P. (1986) *Normative Issues in Social Needs Assessment: a Theoretical Overview*. Faculty Research Paper Series, York, Ontario: York University.

Peterson, C. and McCabe, A. (1983) *Developmental Psycholinguistics: Three Ways of Looking at a Child's Narrative*. New York: Plenum Press.

Pinchbeck, I. and Hewitt, M. (1969) *Children in English Society*, vol. I: *From Tudor Times to the Eighteenth Century*. London: Routledge & Kegan Paul.

—— (1973) *Children in English Society*, vol. II: *From the Eighteenth Century to the Children Act 1948*. London: Routledge & Kegan Paul.

Plant, R., Lessor, H. and Taylor-Gooby, P. (1980) *Political Philosophy and Social Welfare: Essays on the Normative Basis of Welfare Provision*. London: Routledge & Kegan Paul.

Pollock, L. (1983) *Forgotten Children: Parent–Child Relations from 1500 to 1900*. Cambridge: Cambridge University Press.

Priestley, P. (1985) *Victorian Prison Lives: English Prison Biography 1830-1914*. London: Methuen.

Prince, G. (1982) *Narratology: the Form and Functioning of Narrative*. Berlin: Mouton

Propp, V. (1928) *Morphology of the Folk Tale*. American Folklore Society Bibliographical and Special Series, vol. 9 (2nd edn) (ed. L. Wagner, 1968). Austin: University of Texas Press.

Rees, S. (1991) *Achieving Power: Practice and Policy in Social Welfare*. Sydney: Allen & Unwin Pty Ltd.

Richardson, H. (1969) *Adolescent Girls in Approved Schools*. London: Routledge & Kegan Paul.

Richardson, S. (1747/48) *Clarissa or the History of a Young Lady*. Privately printed. For a sound abridgement see that of G. Sherburn (1962), Riverside Editions. Boston MA: Houghton Mifflin.

Ricoeur, P. (1986) *Lectures on Ideology and Utopia*. New York: Columbia University Press.

Rimmon-Kenan, S. (1983) *Narrative Fiction: Contemporary Poetics*. London: Methuen.

Rojek, C., Peacock, G. and Collins, S. (1988) *Social Work and Received Ideas*. London: Routledge.

—— (eds) (1989) *The Haunt of Misery: Critical Essays in Social Work and Helping*. London: Routledge.

Rose, G. (1967) *Schools for Young Offenders*. London: Tavistock.

Rousseau, J.-J. (1762) *Emile or a Treatise on Education* (ed. and trans. by W.H. Payne. London: Sydney Appleton, 1905).

Rushforth, M. (1978) *Committal to Residential Care: a Case Study in Juvenile Justice*. A Scottish Office Social Research Study. Edinburgh: HMSO.

Saussure, F. de (1974) *Course in General Linguistics* (trans. W. Baskin). London: Fontana/Collins.

Schutz, A. (1972) *The Phenomenology of the Social World* (originally published 1932). London: Heinemann Educational Books.

Selden, R. (1985) *A Reader's Guide to Contemporary Literary Theory* (2nd edn). Hemel Hempstead: Harvester Wheatsheaf.

Showalter, E. (1977) *A Literature of Their Own: British Women Novelists from Brontë to Lessing*. Princeton: Princeton University Press.

Sibeon, R. (1991) *Towards a New Sociology of Social Work*. Aldershot: Avebury.

Slater, S. (1967) *Approved School Boy*. London: William Kimber.

Smart, C. (1976) *Women, Crime and Criminology: a Feminist Critique*. London: Routledge & Kegan Paul.

Smart, C. and Sevenhuijsen, S. (eds) (1989) *Child Custody and the Politics of Gender*. London: Routledge.

Smith, G. and May, D. (1980) 'Executing "decisions" in the children's hearings', *Sociology* 14: 581–601.

Soothill, K. and Walby, S. (1991) *Sex Crime in the News*. London: Routledge.

Spark, M. (1988) *Mary Shelley*. London: Constable.

Spicker, P. (1988) *Principles of Social Welfare: an Introduction to Thinking About the Welfare State*. London: Routledge.

Stanzel, F. (1984) *A Theory of Narrative* (trans. C. Goedsche). Cambridge: Cambridge University Press.

Tambling, J. (1991) *Narrative and Ideology*. Milton Keynes: Open University Press.

Thèry, I. (1989) '"The interest of the child" and the regulation of the post-divorce family', in C. Smart and S. Sevenhuijsen (eds), *Child Custody and the Politics of Gender*. London: Routledge.

Thompson, J. (1981) *Critical Hermeneutics: a Study in the Thought of Paul Ricoeur and Jürgen Habermas*. Cambridge: Cambridge University Press.

Thomson, G. (1987) *Needs*. London: Routledge & Kegan Paul.

Timms, N. (1986) 'Value-talk in social work: present character and future improvement', *Issues in Social Work Education* 6: 3–14.

Tobias, J. (1972) *Crime and Industrial Society in the Nineteenth Century*. Harmondsworth: Penguin Books.

Todorov, T. (1977) *The Poetics of Prose* (trans. R. Howard). New York: Cornell University Press.

Utting, W. (1991) *Children in the Public Care*. London: HMSO.

Valk, M. (1983) 'Imaginative literature and social work education: an extended comment on Barker', *Issues in Social Work Education* 3: 17–26.

Von Hirsch, A. (1976) *Doing Justice: the Report of the Committee for the Study of Incarceration*. New York: Hill & Wang.

Warnock, G. (1967) *Contemporary Moral Philosophy*. London: Macmillan.

Webb, D. and Harris, R. (1984) 'Social workers and supervision orders: a case of occupational uncertainty', *British Journal of Social Work* 14: 579–99.

Whan, M. (1979) 'Accounts, narrative and case history', *British Journal of Social Work* 9: 489–99.

Wicker, B. (1975) *The Story-Shaped World: Fiction and Metaphysics: Some Variations on a Theme*. London: The Athlone Press of the University of London.

Williams, R. (1975) *Drama in a Dramatized Society: an Inaugural Lecture*. Cambridge: Cambridge University Press.

Wilson, K. and Ridler, A. (1989) 'Marriage in literature', *British Journal of Social Work* 19: 111–27.

Wilson, T. and Wilson, D. (eds) (1991) *The State and Social Welfare*. London: Longman.

Woolf, V. (1924) *Mr Bennett and Mrs Brown*, Hogarth Essays No. 1. London: Hogarth Press.

—— (1953) *A Writer's Diary: Being Extracts from the Diary of Virginia Woolf* (ed. Leonard Woolf). London: Hogarth Press.

Zander, M. (1980) *The Law-Making Process*. London: Weidenfeld & Nicolson.

Name index

Ackroyd, P. 20
Althusser, L. 22
Anderson, R. 144
Ariès, P. 23, 25, 26, 28, 29, 30, 32, 48, 51, 87, 103, 161
Austen, J. 134

Bagehot, W. 49
Bailey, V. 7
Barnes, J. 20, 181
Barth, K. 60
Barthes, R. 45, 46, 58, 65, 71, 87, 137, 179, 181
Beauvoir, S. de 64
Beckett, S. 60
Bellah, R. 49, 172
Bennett, A. 59, 60, 65, 66
Bennett, J. 102
Benton, T. 36, 41, 42
Blumenthal, G. 24, 95
Boas, G. 25
Bochel, D. 11
Booth, W. 81
Boyne, R. 7, 44, 181
Brecht, B. 59
Buchan, J. 49, 171
Bullock, R. 24, 181
Burney, E. 145

Campbell, A. 130
Campbell, T. 40, 41, 42
Camus, A. 62, 65
Carlen, P. 149, 181
Carpenter, M. 8, 9, 10
Cartland, B. 59
Cavadino, P. 18
Cawson, P. ix, 13, 14, 15, 17, 18, 24, 76
Chatman, S. 179
Clark, G. 17
Clarke, R. 12
Clarke Hall, W. 11
Cohen, S. 5, 101
Collins, J. 59
Connolly, W. 160
Connor, S. 52, 60
Cookson, C. 59
Corelli, M. 64
Cranston, M. 42

Davis, K. 164, 167
Day, S. 9
deMause, L. 32
Derrida, J. 43, 44, 81, 180, 181
Dickens, C. 134
Dingwall, R. 34, 145, 162
Docherty, T. 56
Donzelot, J. 27, 53
Duby, G. 23
Dumas, A. 59
Dworkin, R. 154

Eagleton, T. 31, 179
Eco, U. 57, 60, 64, 181
Eekelaar, J. 36, 88, 144, 145, 162
Eliot, T.S. 60, 66
England, H. 53
Eribon, D. 30

Fielding, H. 118
Fielding, N. 77
Fielder, L. 60

Fleming, I. 64
Flew, A. 40
Fokkema, D. 181
Foucault, M. 7, 30, 43, 50, 63, 66, 100, 180, 181
Fowler, B. 57, 59
Fowles, J. 60, 61
Franklin, B. 17, 29, 162
Fraser, N. 41, 43
Freeman, M. 34, 162
Frost, N. 29

Genette, G. 31, 179
Gewirth, A. 42, 43
Glauberman, S. 85
Godsland, J. 77
Goffman, E. 54, 118, 181
Gramsci, A. 59
Griffin, J. 40

Haimes, E. 53
Hardiker, P. 78
Harding, L. 24, 29, 33, 34, 35, 36, 37, 43, 44, 48, 52, 93, 103, 161
Harland, R. 23, 181
Harris, J. 8
Harris, R. 5, 6, 8, 11, 12, 17, 29, 35, 53, 67, 68, 100, 101, 126, 143, 144, 161
Hawkins, H. 43, 56, 58, 61, 171
Heisenberg, W. K. 59
Henkel, M. 85, 94, 95, 182
Hewitt, M. 24, 32
Heywood, J. 6
Hilgendorf, L. 75, 146, 147, 148, 149
Hoghughi, M. 24
Hoghughi, P. 24
Hohfeld, W. 42
Holloway, J. 181
Holman, R. 34
Holt, J. 17
Homer, 51
Horkheimer, M. 59
Husserl, E. 31
Hutcheon, L. 60, 181

Irvine, E. 53

Jones, P. 42
Joyce, J. 60

Kahan, B. 17, 86, 87
King, M. 150
Kingsley, C. 64
Klein, M. 144
Kleinig, J. 40
Kunne-Ibsch, E. 181

Lacan, J. 43
Lamarque, P. 137
Lévi-Strauss, C. 180
Levy, A. 86, 87
Lodge, D. 60, 181
Lovell, T. 66

McCabe, A. 102
MacIntyre, A. 51, 53, 54, 56, 66, 69, 82, 83, 136, 138, 141, 181
Manton, J. 9
Marlowe, C. 43
Martell, M. ix, 13, 14, 15, 17, 18, 24, 76
Martin, D. 12
Maxwell, R. 13
May, D. 89, 147
Meyer, P. 3
Millham, S. viii, ix, 14, 24, 50, 76, 100, 114
Moi, T. 66
Morris, A. 34
Morris, C. 53
Morris, N. 171

Narayan, K. 58

Oakeshott, M. 43, 78, 160, 169, 179
Olson, C. 60

Packman, J. 6, 50
Page, R. 17
Parker, H. 144
Parton, N. 29, 36
Penz, P. 41
Peterson, C. 102
Pinchbeck, I. 24, 32
Plant, R. 42
Pollock, L. 29, 30, 31, 32, 33, 48, 51, 52
Powell, M. 149, 181
Priestley, P. 9
Prince, G. 82
Propp, V. 57, 181

Radcliffe-Brown, A. R. 180
Rees, S. 181
Richardson, S. 181
Ricoeur, P. 22, 182
Ridler, A. 53
Rimmon-Kenan, S. 57
Rojek, C. viii
Rolph, C. H. 171
Rose, G. 9, 10, 12
Rousseau, J.-J. 25
Rushforth, M. 50

Saussure, F. de 22, 95, 180
Schutz, A. 31
Selden, R. 44, 59, 66, 181
Shakespeare, W. 54
Showalter, E. 66
Sibeon, R. 53
Slater, S. 13
Smart, C. 130
Smith, G. 89, 147
Socrates, 81
Soothill, K. 66
Spark, M. 38
Spicker, P. 42
Stanzel, F. 81
Stein, M. 29
Stoker, B. 64

Tambling, J. 59, 70
Thèry, I. 47
Thompson, J. 182
Thomson, G. 40, 41
Timms, N. 42, 53
Tobias, J. 9
Todorov, T. 181
Tutt, N. 17, 18

Utting, W. 101, 168

Valk, M. 53
Von Hirsch, A. 76

Walby, S. 66
Warhol, A. 60
Warnock, G. 51
Webb, D. 5, 6, 8, 11, 53, 67, 101, 126, 144
Weber, M. 145
Whan, M. 53
Wicker, B. 36, 70, 181
Williams, R. vii, 54
Wilson, K. 53
Woolf, L. 31
Woolf, V. 31, 60, 65, 66

Yeats, W. B. 60

Zander, M. 5
Zola, E. 65

Subject index

absconding 4, 12, 13, 16, 153; *see also* case studies
adolescence 6
Approved Schools 7, 11, 12, 13–14
authorisation 3–4, 38, 77, 80, 81, 83, 88–93, 100, 105, 115, 119, 130, 138–59, 164, 167, 168; and length of hearing 151; and magistrates 155; and renewal applications 80, 156, 166–7; and representation 151–5; and waiting time 150–1

'beyond control' 11
Borstal 7, 12, 14

care: children in 3; nature of 52
'care or protection cases' 49
case studies 102–37
child abuse 28, 29, 32
child care 20–1, 22, 47, 52–3, 76, 84; history of 32; and juvenile justice 4, 13, 25, 47, 65, 77, 141–2; and physical environment 95; policy 6–7, 16, 17, 24, 25, 33–8, 160, 161; *see also* childhood
Child Care Act 1980 18, 173–4
child protection 4, 29, 33, 34, 161; and the role of the court 141
childhood 7–8, 22, 49, 50, 52, 88, 93, 161, 162, 172; concept of 25, 32, 49; and family 23, 24; history of 25–33; and state 23
Children Act 1908 9
Children Act 1989 18, 36, 145, 164, 175–6, 180
Children and Young Persons Act 1933 3, 10–11, 14, 77
Children and Young Persons Act 1969 11–12
Children's Legal Centre 17, 18, 24, 76, 83, 86, 87, 100
citizenship: and children 8, 24, 162
community homes 13
community service orders 5
courts: and children's rights 80, 138, 139, 140, 141, 143, 144; and family 23–4; and lawyers 68–9; and secure accommodation 20, 104, 138–59, 164, 165, 166, 167; and social workers 68–9, 164; *see also* juvenile court, magistrates
crime 6, 7, 10, 12, 49, 162; and social need 13
Criminal Justice Act 1991 177–8, 180, 182
Criminal Justice Bill 1982 18
criminality 12, 50; and deprivation 62
criteria: and secure accommodation 3–4, 14, 17–18, 90–3, 127, 152, 153–4
culture 52, 54, 59, 62; *see also* literature
Curtis Report 12

decarceration 16
decision making 46, 52–3, 68, 76, 79, 83, 86–7, 88–93, 139–40, 145, 147, 149, 156, 164, 165–6; *see also* case studies
delinquency *see* juvenile delinquency
discharge: from secure accommodation 120–3, 157–9, 167, 169

discourse 21, 31, 40, 43, 45, 50, 52, 53, 69, 95, 107
drama: in social work 51–71
duties: children's 162

European Convention on Human Rights 18, 166
'experts': as advisers 68–9; child-care 52–3; and decision making 68; role of 4, 5, 27, 50, 54, 56, 61, 65, 67–70; *see also* case studies, professionals, social workers

family 5, 8, 11, 19, 33, 34, 36, 50, 59, 70, 172; and control of children 21, 23, 24, 25–6; history of 25–33, 51–2; and the state 5, 11, 20–48, 160–2, 164
Franklin Report 1951 12

gender: bias 126–34
girls: and secure accommodation 126–34
Gladstone Report 1895 10
Guardian *ad litem*: role of 145–6, 148, 158, 166

Health and Social Services and Social Security Adjudications Bill 1983 18
Howard Association 11
Howard League for Penal Reform 16
human rights 18

industrial schools 8–11
Industrial Schools Act 1857 9
inspection: of secure accommodation 93–5
'interest of the child' 46–7, 78
interests 4–5, 7, 24, 34, 38, 39, 41–2, 43, 45, 47, 52, 75, 76, 88, 91, 114, 136, 138, 139, 145, 146, 148, 162

juvenile court: and relationship with social services departments 139, 140–1; role of 3, 12, 18, 90; *see also* courts, magistrates
juvenile delinquency 5, 6–12, 50, 65, 70, 162, 171–2; and adult crime 49
juvenile delinquents 6; management of 49, 75

Kahan Report 1979 17

labelling 108
language 22, 51; of social workers 56
law 21, 28, 68, 160, 162
literature 51–71, 136–7
local authorities: and inspection of secure accommodation 93–5; and juvenile courts 139, 140–1; and policy documents 84; and secure accommodation 3, 4, 15–16, 17, 18, 75, 76, 77–8, 80, 83–4, 88, 90–3, 139–40, 143, 144, 145, 148, 165, 166, 169; *see also* decision making
logocentrism, 44–5, 48, 103

magistrates: role of 139–40, 145, 147, 149, 155, 156; training of 143–4, 166–7; *see also* courts
Magistrates Association 16
'medical model' 107–8

narrative: in social work 51–71, 81–2, 102–3, 104, 163, 179
National Association for the Care and Resettlement of Offenders 18
National Association of Young People in Care 17
needs 4–5, 7, 11, 13, 24, 38–41, 43, 46–7, 50, 52, 75, 76, 78, 88, 91, 93, 100, 114, 125, 136, 138, 139, 145, 146, 148, 162
needy children 5, 6, 9, 11–12, 19, 49

parents *see* family
phenomenology 31, 51, 70
'pindown' 86–7
Police Federation 16
Prevention of Cruelty to and Protection of Children Act 1889 28
prisons 5, 10; and children 76–7
professionals: role of 103, 107, 116, 139, 141, 143, 147, 149, 158, 161–2, 163; *see also* case studies, experts, social workers
psychiatrist: role of 107, 116
public: protection of 104
punishment 7, 11, 12, 27; and secure accommodation 50, 144

Radical Alternatives to Prison 16
reformatory schools 8, 9–10, 11
Reformatory Schools Amendment Act 1899 9
Regional Youth Treatment Centres 15
remand: children on 3, 76–7, 123–6; *see also* case study 123–6
renewal applications 80, 156, 166–7
Report of the Children Committee 1946 12
Report of the Departmental Committee on Reformatory and Industrial Schools 1896 10
Report of the Enquiry into the Disturbance at Carlton School 1959 13–14
Report of the Home Office Working Party on Closed and Other Special Facilities in Approved Schools 1960 14
rights: children's 4–5, 7, 16, 17, 24, 28, 33, 34, 35, 38, 39, 42–3, 47, 52, 69, 76, 80, 88, 91, 93, 114, 125, 136, 138, 139, 141, 143, 144, 145, 146, 148, 162; human 42; natural 42; parents' 33, 34, 36

secure accommodation: and authorisation 3–4; and care 4; and child care 20–1; and control 4; and courts 20, 104, 138–59, 164, 165, 166, 167; criteria for 3–4, 14, 17–18, 90–3, 152, 153–4; discharge from 120–3, 157–9, 167, 169; and finance 97; and girls 126–34; guidelines for 17; historical background of 6, 12–19, 75–7; and increase in 169–70; and independent review 165–6; inspection of 93–5; and length of time in 4; and locality 97; nature of 4, 5, 24, 39, 45, 50, 52, 71, 96–8, 144, 162–3, 164, 170, 171–2; and planning 97; and policy implementation 5; and relations between state, family and child 20–48; and '72-hour rule' 81, 83–8, 99, 100; and 6-month renewal 167; types of 99; use of 3, 17–21, 29, 83–8, 99–100, 169–70; *see also* local authorities, secure units
secure units 14–15, 76, 108; and expenditure 76; inspection of 17; *see also* secure accommodation
security 38, 40, 86
self-determination 42, 71, 98
Social Services Inspectorate (SSI) 93–4, 95, 166
social work 53, 150; and drama 51–71; as a dramatic intervention 53, 54–5; as narrative 51–71, 81–2, 102–3, 104, 163, 179
Social Work Advisory Service (SWAS) 94, 95
social workers 50, 53, 61, 66, 71, 76, 103, 141, 145–6, 147–8, 156, 158; and courts 68–9, 164; and decision making 91–2; and drama 51–71; and language 56; and power 36, 38, 41; *see also* case studies, 'experts', professionals
solicitors 68–9, 141, 144, 146–7, 149–50, 151–5, 158, 168
staff 87, 101, 168–9; comments of 95–8; management of 84–5; support of 84-5; and training 84–6, 168–9
state 6–7, 70, 91, 156, 172; and the child 23, 47, 52, 87; and the family 5, 11, 20–48, 87, 93, 160–2, 164
symbolic interactionism 54

tabloid press 66–7
therapy: use of 4, 14, 108–9, 117–19, 168; *see also* treatment
training: of magistrates 143–4, 166–7; of staff 84–6, 168–9
treatment 5, 14, 138–9, 156; *see also* therapy

Unruly Certificates 140, 144

'value-perspectives' 24, 29, 33–8, 43, 44, 48, 103, 161
voluntarism 7, 49, 64

welfare of the child 11, 144

Youthful Offenders Act 1854 9